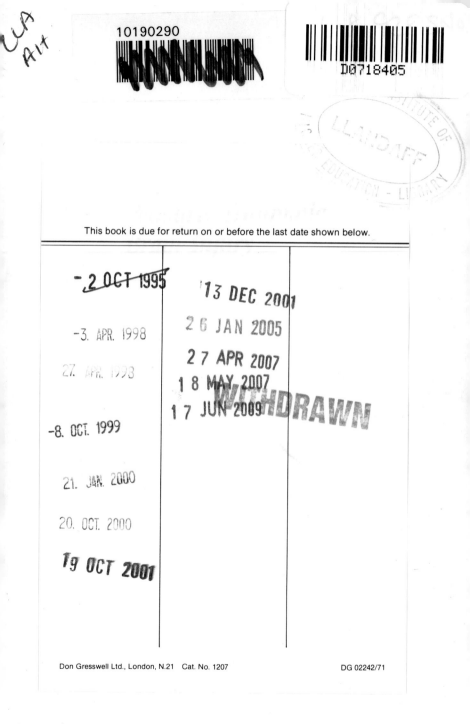

Developmental Clinical Psychology and Psychiatry Series

Series Editor: Alan E. Kazdin, Yale University

Recent volumes in this series . . .

Pediatric Traumatic Brain Injury

Jeffrey H. Snow
Stephen R. Hooper

Volume 31.
Developmental Clinical Psychology and Psychiatry

 SAGE Publications
International Educational and Professional Publisher
Thousand Oaks   London   New Delhi

For information address:

 SAGE Publications, Inc.
2455 Teller Road
Thousand Oaks, California 91320

SAGE Publications Ltd.
6 Bonhill Street
London EC2A 4PU
United Kingdom

SAGE Publications India Pvt. Ltd.
M-32 Market
Greater Kailash I
New Delhi 110 048 India

Printed in the United States of America

Library of Congress Cataloging-in-Publication Data

Snow, Jeffrey H.
    Pediatric traumatic brain injury / Jeffrey H. Snow, Stephen R. Hooper.
    p. cm. — (Developmental clinical psychology and psychiatry; v. 31)
    Includes bibliographical references and index.
    ISBN 0-8039-5181-7 (cloth). — ISBN 0-8039-5182-5 (pbk.)
    1. Brain-damaged children. I. Hooper, Stephen R. II. Title. III. Series.
    [DNLM: 1. Brain Injuries—in infancy & childhood. 2. Brain Injuries—in adolescence. W1 DE997NC v. 31 1994 / WS 340 S674p 1994]
RJ496.B7S66 1994
618.92'8—dc20
DNLM/DLC   94-19745

94 95 96 97 98 10 9 8 7 6 5 4 3 2 1

Sage Production Editor: Diane S. Foster

To Laura, Christopher, and Thomas for their love and support. JHS

To Mary for her constant love and support in all of my academic pursuits, and to Lindsay and Madeline for putting these pursuits into their proper perspective. SRH

CONTENTS

Part III: Assessment and Treatment

Part IV: Postscript

SERIES EDITOR'S INTRODUCTION

Interest in child development and adjustment is by no means new. Yet, only recently has the study of children benefited from advances in both clinical and scientific research. Advances in the social and biological sciences; the emergence of disciplines and subdisciplines that focus exclusively on childhood and adolescence; and greater appreciation of the impact of such influences as the family, peers, and school have helped accelerate research on developmental psychopathology. Apart from interest in the study of child development and adjustment for its own sake, the need to address clinical problems of adulthood naturally draws one to investigate precursors in childhood and adolescence.

Within a relatively brief period, the study of psychopathology among children and adolescents has proliferated considerably. Several different professional journals, annual book series, and handbooks devoted entirely to the study of children and adolescents and their adjustment document the proliferation of work in the field. Nevertheless, there is a paucity of resource material that presents information in an authoritative, systematic, and disseminable fashion. There is a need within the field to convey the latest developments and to represent different disciplines, approaches, and conceptual views to the topics of childhood and adolescent adjustment and maladjustment.

The Sage Series, *Developmental Clinical Psychology and Psychiatry,* is designed to serve uniquely several needs of the field. The series encompasses individual monographs prepared by experts in the fields of clinical child psychology, child psychiatry, child development, and related disciplines. The primary focus is on developmental psychopathology which refers broadly here to the diagnosis, assessment, treatment, and prevention of problems that arise in the period from infancy through adolescence. A working assumption of the series is that understanding, identifying, and treating problems of youth must draw on multiple disciplines and diverse views within a given discipline.

The task for individual contributors is to present the latest theory and research on various topics including specific types of dysfunction, diagnostic and treatment approaches, and special problems that affect adjustment. Core topics within clinical work are addressed by the series. Authors are asked to bridge potential theory, research, and clinical practice, and to outline the current status and future directions. The goals of the series and the tasks presented to individual contributors are demanding. We have been extremely fortunate in recruiting leaders in the fields who have been able to translate their recognized scholarship and expertise into highly readable works on contemporary topics.

Traumatic brain injury in children and adolescents represents a set of dysfunctions with broad impact and consequences for the individual, family, and society at large. In the present monograph, Drs. Jeffrey H. Snow and Stephen R. Hooper convey advances in our understanding of different types of injuries, how they occur, the scope of impairment to which they can lead, and the factors that influence their outcomes. The scope of the problem, variations, in incidence and prevalence of injury by child age and sex, and the impact of premorbid functioning on outcomes are carefully presented. The detailed discussion of the range of outcomes following brain injury related to cognitive (e.g., academic performance and mental abilities) and psychosocial functioning (e.g., psychiatric disorders and varied emotional and behavioral problems) is particularly noteworthy. Measurement of neurological status (e.g., imaging techniques, neuropsychological testing) and utilization of test information for diagnosis are illustrated. Alternative interventions such as those available in the schools as well as for the family are also presented. The book conveys well the relation between brain injury and psychosocial functioning and the current status of assessment and intervention to aid youth with such injuries. Hence, in a very important way, this book helps to elaborate the complex and reciprocal relations between psychological and neurological functioning and how both influence adjustment and adaptive functioning.

—Alan E. Kazdin, Ph.D.

PREFACE

This volume is designed to provide an introduction to pediatric traumatic brain injury (TBI). Unfortunately, TBI continues to occur all too frequently, and negatively impacts the lives of children, adolescents, and their family members. On a more positive note, research efforts have begun to advance our knowledge of the cognitive and behavioral consequences of traumatic head injuries. Services for TBI children and adolescents continue to expand, and as a result, increasing numbers of professionals are becoming involved with this group.

Traumatically brain-injured victims can be particularly challenging. These individuals are not only subjected to potential long-standing cognitive and behavioral sequelae, but also must deal with a traumatic incident that often results in lengthy hospital stays. Reintegration to home, community, and school settings can be problematic and places a great deal of stress on all involved. It is critical that professionals working with children and adolescents who have sustained a TBI have a broad-based understanding of the neurological, cognitive, and emotional/behavioral aspects of this clinical population.

This volume is designed to be an introductory text for professionals who may work with children and adolescents with traumatic brain injuries. The first part addresses some basics, with specific chapters devoted to definitional issues, epidemiology of acquired brain injuries, and neurological principles. The chapter on neurological foundations in TBI will be especially pertinent to a wide variety of professionals not having such information in their training backgrounds; however, it is important to note that the neurological bases of TBI go well beyond what is presented in this chapter. Nonetheless, the basic neurological issues in TBI are addressed, and ample references are provided for readers who may want more.

The second part of this book contains two chapters: one addressing neuro-pathological mechanisms and another relating current information on what is known about ultimate outcomes from a TBI. The chapter on mechanisms provides information on the various neurological factors that can come into play; the outcome chapter provides information via a construct-driven approach. Issues related to recovery and cognitive/psychosocial outcomes are discussed.

The third part focuses on assessment and intervention. Chapters cover topics such as neurodiagnostic techniques and neuropsychological assessment. Evaluation of behavior and social-emotional functions also is discussed. This part concludes with a chapter reviewing selected intervention strategies and an illustrative case study. The postscript reviews pertinent issues addressed in this volume.

Overall, the volume represents a brief overview of theoretical as well as practical considerations relevant to TBI. The content of this volume is largely focused on TBI among school-aged children, adolescents, and to some extent preschool-aged children. This is not to deny the importance of issues relevant to infants and very young children; rather, sufficient discussion of early-stage development and effects of traumatic brain injury calls for a separate volume to be devoted to such a topic.

This volume is designed for students and professionals in the areas of clinical psychology, school psychology, education, and other disciplines where direct contact with TBI children/adolescents is possible through their clinical practice. Clinical and research activities in this area continue to expand, yet considerable work is still needed. With these efforts, we should continue to increase our understanding of the cognitive/behavioral consequences of TBI, as well as more effectively meet the needs of these children and adolescents. We hope that this introductory volume makes a contribution to these efforts.

Part I

Foundations

1

DEFINITIONAL ISSUES AND EPIDEMIOLOGICAL CHARACTERISTICS

Neurological involvement of any kind can have a significant impact on the overall functioning of a child or adolescent. This is especially possible in the case of traumatic brain injury (TBI), where the sudden nature of the injury and its severity can alter the developmental progression, expectations, and environmental arena of an individual forever. Such a brain injury also can have devastating effects on family functioning (D. A. Martin, 1990). Recognizing the possible impact that a TBI can have on an individual will assist the child psychologist and other child practitioners in developing assessment, treatment, and tracking programs for these individuals; however, most child professionals are ill prepared to manage such cases.

Despite a historic shortage of formal training opportunities on TBI in most traditional clinical, school, and counseling psychology training programs, as well as in other pediatric disciplines (e.g., social work, special education), recent changes in federal legislation governing special education services have stimulated more active interest in this population. Consequently, although children and adolescents who have sustained traumatic brain injuries have been around forever, it would seem that increased interest will be devoted to this population over the next decade. Furthermore, it has been only within the last two decades or so that our knowledge about child and adolescent TBI has begun to emerge. In this chapter, we will discuss definitional issues related to traumatic brain injury. Issues related to epidemiology, specific causes of TBI, and associated risk factors for children and adolescents also will be presented.

DEFINITIONAL ISSUES

The National Head Injury Foundation (NHIF, 1985) defines a traumatic brain injury as "an insult to the brain, not of a degenerative or congenital nature, but caused by an external force, that may produce a diminished or altered state of consciousness." Although basic by design, this definition addresses most of the core issues pertinent to operationalizing traumatic brain injury. First, this definition states that a TBI must be caused by an external force. Although a brain insult can occur via any number of neurological mechanisms, such as a cerebrovascular accident, various kinds of tumors, and epileptogenic brain activity, it is important to recognize that a TBI arises only in the case where an external force is involved. This is consistent with the specialized field of trauma medicine. At the same time, it is important to note that this "external force" does not necessarily have to be a direct blow to the head. The effects of acceleration-deceleration, as can be seen in the case of a shaken infant or a motor vehicle accident, may be the external force that creates the brain injury without any physical contact actually occurring (Jennett, 1986). Second, the definition addresses the issue of change in functioning when compared to preinjury status. This is extremely important with respect to the assessment and treatment of individuals who have sustained a traumatic brain injury.

One of the most recent attempts to operationalize traumatic brain injury has come from the Individuals With Disabilities Education Act (IDEA; U.S. Office of Education, 1990). An interagency committee composed of representatives from the National Head Injury Foundation (NHIF), Office of Special Education and Rehabilitation Services (OSERS), Council of State Administrators of Vocational Rehabilitation (CSAVR), and National Association of State Directors of Special Education (NASDSE) was organized in 1985 to promote the recognition and expansion of services to individuals who had sustained traumatic brain injuries. It was the efforts of this collaborative group that spawned the IDEA legislation. The IDEA legislation, formerly known as the Education of the Handicapped Act, was signed into law in the fall of 1990 and amended the definition of children with disabilities to include children with brain injuries. In addition, this legislation has mandated TBI as a new exceptional children classification. This definition reads as follows (Federal Register, 1992, p. 44842):

> Traumatic brain injury means an acquired injury to the brain caused by an external physical force, resulting in total or partial functional disability or psychosocial impairment, or both, that adversely affects a child's educational performance. The term applies to open or closed head injuries resulting in impairments in one or more areas, such as cognition; language; memory; attention; reasoning; abstract thinking; judgment; problem-solving; sensory, perceptual and motor abilities; psychosocial behavior, physical functions; information processing; and speech. The term does not apply to brain injuries that are congenital or degenerative, or brain injuries induced by birth trauma.

Similar to its predecessor from the NHIF, this federal definition includes the issues of injury mechanism as well as attempts to describe the "altered state of consciousness" in more detail (e.g., impairments in language, memory, etc.).

These definitional efforts are noteworthy in paving the way for increased recognition of issues relevant to the child and adolescent with TBI. Furthermore, with the IDEA legislation, not only will these individuals be eligible for increased services, particularly in the public school setting, but assessment and treatment strategies for this population likely will become more refined and clinically relevant.

Despite these efforts, however, the definitions remain simplistic with respect to addressing the myriad of issues involved in defining traumatic brain injury. Indeed, Levin, Benton, and Grossman (1982) reviewed several systematic attempts to classify different types of traumatic injuries, but each has been challenged on its ability to reflect actual brain injury, particularly in mild cases. At present, there appear to be at least three core issues pertinent to the definition of a traumatic brain injury: an alteration in the level of consciousness; the degree of posttraumatic amnesia (PTA); and the presence of neurophysiological, neuroanatomical, and/or some other type of physical damage (Bigler, 1990).

Alteration in the Level of Consciousness

As noted in the NHIF and federal definitions of TBI, an altered state of consciousness is one of the key features cited. Although it is recognized that such changes can be common sequelae of most traumatic brain injuries, variants to this corollary are quite common. For example, such alterations do not always appear with some brain injuries (Jennett, 1986),

TABLE 1.1 Items and Categories on the Glasgow Coma Scale

Eye Openings	Best Verbal Response	Best Motor·Response
4. Spontaneous	5. Oriented	6. Responds to verbal
3. Nonspecific	4. Confusion,	commands
reaction to speech	disorientation	5. Localized movement to
2. Response to	3. No sustained or coherent	terminate painful stimulus
painful stimulus	conversation	4. Withdrawal from painful
1. No response	2. No recognizable words	stimulus
	1. No response	3. Decorticate posture
		2. Decerebrate posture
		1. No response

SOURCE: Adapted from Teasdale and Jennett (1974).

as can be the case with selected types of focal injuries, and in other cases the alterations may be temporally delayed (e.g., edema, hematoma). Conversely, a brief alteration in the state of consciousness with quick and total recovery of functioning, as might be seen in a concussion (Bakay & Glasauer, 1980), may not be sufficient to invoke the inference of a traumatic brain injury. Consequently, care should be taken when making a direct linkage between the presence/absence of an altered state of consciousness and a resultant brain injury.

In light of these cautionary notes, several attempts have been advanced to quantify the relevant level of consciousness. Over 20 years ago Teasdale and Jennett (1974) developed the Glasgow Coma Scale (GCS) (Table 1.1). The GCS is a clinician rating scale designed to evaluate three key aspects of consciousness: the amount of stimulation to create an eye opening, the best verbal response, and the best motor response. Ratings range from a low score of 3 to a high score of 15. In general, a GCS score of 8 or less is indicative of a severe brain injury, scores of 9 through 12 reflect a moderate level of severity, and scores of 13 to 14 indicate a mild brain injury. A score of 15 likely reflects the lack of an altered state of consciousness. The GCS has been used successfully in emergency rooms and has offered some index of the degree of severity (Bond, 1983). It also has provided some clues with respect to prognosis (Heiden, Small, Caton, Weiss, & Kurtze, 1983).

Although the GCS has been used for individuals ranging in age from 3 years through adulthood, other adaptations of the GCS have been devel-

TABLE 1.2 Items and Categories on the Children's Coma Scale

Eye Openings	Best Motor Response	Best Behavior Response
4. Spontaneous	6. Responds to verbal commands	5. Smiles, oriented to sound, interacts, follows objects
3. Nonspecific reaction to speech	5. Localized movement to terminate painful stimulus	4. Consolable crying, but inappropriate interactions
2. Response to painful stimulus	4. Withdrawal from painful stimulus	3. Inconsistently consolable, moaning
1. No response	3. Decorticate posture	2. Inconsolable, restless, and irritable
	2. Decerebrate posture	1. No response
	1. No response	

SOURCE: Adapted from Hahn et al. (1988).

oped specifically for children (Morray, Tyler, Jones, Stuntz, & Lemire, 1984; Simpson & Reilly, 1982). For example, similar to the GCS, the Pediatric Coma Scale (Simpson & Reilly, 1982) includes the child's best response in motor, verbal, and eyes open modalities. The best responses are rated and then added together to gain a total score. This total score is then compared against an age-based normal aggregate standard. Similarly, the Children's Coma Scale (Hahn et al., 1988) was developed for children under the age of 3 years, and rates the child's best performance in eyes open, motor, and behavioral responses categories (Table 1.2).

Degree of Posttraumatic Amnesia

The degree of posttraumatic amnesia (PTA) also has been invoked as a useful mechanism for defining the severity of a TBI (Brooks, 1983). PTA, or anterograde amnesia, is the amount of time following a brain injury that an individual experiences difficulties learning and retaining new information. PTA is the time following an injury when the individual is conscious and functioning (i.e., not comatose) and capable of responding in a relatively reliable manner. PTA ends when the individual's continuous memories are restored (Rosen & Gerring, 1986). Although there may be significant retrograde amnesia as well (i.e., lack of recall for events prior to the accident), PTA has been deemed useful for defining the severity of a TBI. This distinction is graphically depicted in Figure 1.1. Brooks (1983) noted that a severe PTA of at least one week or more has been related to poorer outcome, particularly in the cognitive and psychosocial domains.

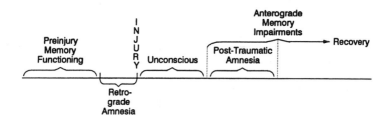

Figure 1.1. Schematic Representation Distinguishing Retrograde Amnesia, Posttraumatic Amnesia, and Anterograde Amnesia.
SOURCE: Ruff et al. (1989). Reprinted with permission.

There also have been several attempts to quantify the degree of PTA. Russell (1971) described a PTA of less than 5 minutes as very mild, 5 minutes to 1 hour as mild, 1 to 24 hours as moderate, 1 to 7 days as severe, and beyond 7 days as very severe. Similarly, Levin, O'Donnell, and Grossman (1979) developed the Galveston Orientation and Amnesia Test (GOAT) to assist in this endeavor. The GOAT is a 10-item bedside test of orientation and continuous memory that is administered serially to document the return of these functions. Ewing-Cobbs, Levin, Fletcher, Miner, and Eisenberg (1990) modified this for children to produce the Children's Orientation and Amnesia Test (COAT). The COAT can be given to children aged 3 through 15. The ability of these procedures to be administered serially is important in that individuals with severe PTA can still exhibit islands of memory, and the ongoing nature of this testing will assist in identifying the deficits that do exist.

Presence of Physical Damage

A final issue that must be included in conceptualizing a definition of TBI is whether there is any actual physical damage that can be identified in the brain. This physical damage can be in the form of neurophysiological evidence, as can be uncovered with electroencephalographic assessment strategies; neuroanatomical evidence, as depicted with a variety of neuroimaging procedures such as computerized axial tomography (CT scan), magnetic resonance imaging (MRI), or functional magnetic resonance; and/or in the form of direct physical examination (e.g., neuropsychological deficits, speech and language impediments, hemiparesis, cortical blindness).

Findings from these procedures, when used jointly with the presence of PTA and the degree of consciousness, offer a more comprehensive, multidimensional approach to defining TBI. Precise descriptions of these neurophysiological and neuroimaging procedures may be obtained via a variety of technical resources (e.g., Bigler, in press; Duffy & McAnulty, 1985).

EPIDEMIOLOGICAL CHARACTERISTICS

The complexity of the definitional issues relevant to TBI is also of concern in the epidemiology of TBI in children and adolescents. In fact, Kraus (1987) cited the lack of consistency across studies in the definition of a head injury and noted how this has hindered the ascertainment of an accurate estimate of TBI cases. For example, facial lacerations and bruises have been lumped under the category of head injury, although little evidence existed with respect to the presence of a brain injury in such cases. Furthermore, Goldstein and Levin (1987) noted that many potential brain injuries have been diagnosed by the cause (e.g., fall, motor vehicle accident), rather than by the nature of the injury. These investigators also cited the pitfalls attached to developing incidence estimates based on hospital admission records and telephone surveys. These methodological issues contribute to the difficulties in gaining an accurate estimate of the incidence and prevalence of traumatic brain injury in children and adolescents.

Nonetheless, it has been estimated that traumatic brain injury represents one of the most frequent neurological conditions that result in hospitalization of children and adolescents under 19 years of age (Field, 1976), with some estimates suggesting that TBI accounts for approximately 4% of hospital admissions (North, 1976). Furthermore, TBI is a major contribution to mortality and morbidity in children and adolescents (Fletcher, Ewing-Cobbs, McLaughlin, & Levin, 1985; Frankowski, 1985; Levin et al., 1982). In general, TBI represents a major health problem because it is the leading cause of death or permanent disability in children and adolescents (Guyer & Ellers, 1990).

Incidence Rates and Related Factors

To date, there have been several epidemiological studies conducted to examine specific issues pertinent to traumatic brain injury (e.g., Annegers, 1983; Guyer & Ellers, 1990; Hahn et al., 1988; Ivan, Choo, & Ventureya,

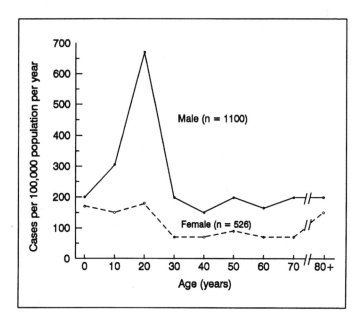

Figure 1.2. Incidence Rates of Head Trauma in Olmsted County, Minnesota, 1964-1974.

SOURCE: Annegers, Grabow, Kurland, and Laws (1980). Reprinted with permission.

1983; Kraus, 1987; Kraus, Fife, Cox, Ramstein, & Conroy, 1986). Annegers, Grabow, Kurland, and Laws (1980) conducted one of the first epidemiological studies that employed clear diagnostic criteria to ascertain incidence rates. Using the population in Olmsted County, Minnesota, these investigators obtained an overall incidence rate of 386 per 100,000, with males (270/100,000) showing over a 2:1 ratio when compared to females (116/100,000). In addition to the gender differences, specific age trends also were observed in the data. Specifically, Annegers et al. (1980) found that the incidence of TBI increased significantly in the 15-to-24 age range, particularly for males. More specifically, males showed a heightened rate from ages 5 to 25 years whereas females demonstrated a decline from age 3 years through age 15 years. There also were secondary peaks during infancy and after age 70. These trends can be seen in Figure 1.2.

Similar trends were obtained by Kraus et al. (1984) in their study of medical records of patients who died or who were admitted to San Diego

County Hospital in 1981. When taken together, Goldstein and Levin (1987) and Frankowski, Annegers, and Whitman (1985) reported incidence rates of 150/100,000 for ages birth to 4 years; 550/100,000 for ages 15 to 19; 160/100,000 around age 50; and 200/100,000 for age 65 and beyond.

Focusing on pediatric head injury (i.e., ages birth to 14 years), Annegers (1983) reported an incidence rate of 220/100,000. This was consistent with the 230/100,000 rate reported by Kalsbeek, McLaurin, Harris, and Miller (1980), and the 185/100,000 rated provided by Kraus et al. (1986). Kraus, Rock, and Hemyari (1990) also reported different incidence rates for different degrees of TBI severity in children ranging in age from birth to age 15. These rates indicated that about 5% of TBI's are fatal, whereas 6%, 8%, and 81% were described as severe, moderate, and mild, respectively.

Furthermore, when pediatric mortality rates were examined for TBI, they were significantly greater than the second major cause of pediatric death—leukemia. Jennett and Teasdale (1981) noted a lower mortality rate for children compared to adults, perhaps because of associated medical conditions in adults and/or the observation that children may be more readily admitted to a hospital following such a trauma (Cooper, 1982). Gender differences also were observed, with males having about a fourfold risk of death from a TBI over females (Moyes, 1980).

In addition to differences reported in the age, gender, and severity of the TBI, information has begun to emerge with respect to the impact of race, socioeconomic status, and time of day or year on the incidence rates of TBI. Studies conducted by Kraus (1987), Rivara and Mueller (1986), and Cooper, Tabaddor, Hauser, Schulman, Feiner, and Factor (1983) revealed a higher rate of TBI in minority populations when compared to whites. As Fennell and Mickle (1992) noted, however, these studies generally failed to take into account the effects of socioeconomic status on the incidence rates. In fact, in his review of major epidemiological efforts in TBI, Kraus (1987) reported that the highest rates of TBI were observed in sociocultural groups with the lowest median income, suggesting that these socioeconomic factors should be considered when exploring incidence rates of TBI.

Temporal fluctuations also have been reported with respect to the epidemiology of pediatric TBI. These fluctuations have been seen with respect to specific times of the day (Levin et al., 1982), specific days (Edna, 1987), and specific seasons of the year, depending on region of the country (Klauber et al., 1981). For example, the likelihood of a child or adolescent incurring a TBI increases from the time that school ends to the time they go to bed (Levin et al., 1982). Falls are most likely to occur between noon and 6 p.m., and motor vehicle accidents between 6 p.m. and 9 p.m. (Jagger, Levine, Jane, & Rimel, 1984). Traumatic brain injuries tend to occur with a higher frequency on weekends, with peak days being Friday and Saturday (Edna, 1987; Klonoff & Thompson, 1969). Geographically, where weather patterns are more stable, stable rates of TBI are observed (Klauber et al., 1981); however, in regions of the country where more variable weather patterns are observed, an increased rate of traumatic brain injuries is observed during the spring and summer months (Edna, 1987).

Selected risk factors also have been discussed that might increase the chance of a traumatic brain injury in selected populations of children and adolescents. For example, Rutter, Chadwick, Shaffer, and Brown (1980) noted that these individuals may not represent a random cut of the general population. Their mildly injured group of children showed a higher rate of psychosocial problems, but these problems likely preceded the TBI. Similarly, Craft, Shaw, and Cartlidge (1972) found an increased rate of teacher-reported problems, including hyperactivity, depression, and antisocial behaviors which, again, predated the brain injury. Premorbid developmental difficulties and specific learning problems (Klonoff & Paris, 1974), language problems (Mahoney et al., 1983), and lower academic achievement (Chadwick, Rutter, Brown, Shaffer, & Traub, 1981) also have been reported for pediatric traumatic brain injury samples.

Finally, recent evidence does suggest that an individual who sustains a traumatic brain injury is at increased risk, perhaps because of the sequelae incurred from the first TBI, for sustaining a second brain injury. Annegers et al. (1980) reported that this risk was age related, with risk being increased twofold under age 14 years, threefold between the ages of 15 and 24 years, and fivefold after age 25. Males also had twice the likelihood of sustaining a second TBI as females.

Major Causes of TBI
in Children and Adolescents

Along with factors related to gender, race, socioeconomic status, chronological age, and temporal variations, specific causes for traumatic brain injuries have been described. For example, accidents in the home account for the major number of head injuries in preschool children, although child abuse is rapidly gaining in this age group (Christoffel, 1990). Rivara

TABLE 1.3 Percentages of Children in Houston and Galveston Sustaining Head Trauma From Different Causes

Cause	Under 1 (n = 68)	1-4 (n = 221)	Age (years) 5-9 (n = 183)	10-14 (n = 134)	15-19 (n = 517)
Motor Vehicle Accident	26.0	17.2	25.7	37.3	51.8
Motorcycle	—	0.5	1.6	0.7	8.7
Pedestrian	1.5	20.4	39.3	15.7	6.0
Bicycle	—	0.9	9.3	9.0	1.9
Fall	61.8	50.7	18.6	20.1	9.7
Gunshot Wound	1.5	2.3	—	4.5	7.9
Assault	5.9	2.7	0.5	3.0	8.5
Other	3.3	5.3	5.0	9.7	5.5
Total	100.0	100.0	100.0	100.0	100.0

SOURCE: Taken from Frankowski, R. F. (1985). Head injury mortality in urban populations and its relation to the injured child. In Brooks, B. F. (Ed.), *The Injured Child*. Austin: University of Texas Press. With permission.

(1984) observed that infants and preschoolers may be at risk for head versus trunk and extremity injuries due to the disproportionate size of an infant's head and a higher center of gravity. Falls, pedestrian-motor vehicle accidents, bicycle-motor vehicle accidents, and sporting activities comprise the majority of mild TBI in school-aged children (Comninos, 1979; Klauber et al., 1981; Klonoff, 1971), whereas motor vehicle accidents cause the majority of severe TBI cases for older children and adults (Rutter et al., 1980). Similar findings are reported by Frankowski (1985) and can be seen in Table 1.3.

In general, the cause of TBI tends to change with age and may contribute to the actual pathophysiology of the TBI in question. For example, more severe brain injuries tend to be incurred by older adolescents and adults secondary to high-speed motor vehicle accidents. In contrast, Kalsbeek et al. (1980) have reported that a similar level of severity in a TBI incurred from a fall may be created by compression of cortical and subcortical regions secondary to intracerebral hematoma as opposed to frank brain damage. Similarly, a TBI resulting from a fall may develop intracranial hematomas, whereas a TBI resulting from a motor vehicle accident more likely results in concussion (DiRocco & Velardi, 1986).

SUMMARY

In this chapter, we have presented some of the key background components to understanding the scope of traumatic brain injury in children and adolescents. As can be seen, the issue of defining TBI is not a simple matter of determining whether a child has received a significant blow to the head. The multiple dimensions that need to be taken into consideration in determining whether a significant brain injury has occurred and the severity of that injury contribute to a complex array of variables for clinical considerations.

These issues spill over into the determination of epidemiological features associated with TBI. It will be important for the child psychologist to be cognizant of these features when confronted with a clinical situation in which a traumatic brain injury might have occurred in a child or adolescent patient. In general, it is clear that TBI is not randomly distributed with respect to chronological age, gender, premorbid learning and personality characteristics, and perhaps race and socioeconomic status. It will be important for these issues to be kept in mind as other aspects of TBI are presented in following chapters.

2

NEUROLOGICAL FOUNDATIONS IN TRAUMATIC BRAIN INJURY

From Chapter 1, it should be clear that traumatic brain injury can be much more complex than a bump on the head and/or a brief loss of consciousness. The relatively frequent occurrence of traumatic brain injuries makes this group of disorders a major health concern and has prompted the development of many guidelines as well as legislation for safety and prevention (e.g., seat belt and child safety seat laws, bicycle and motorcycle helmet use, child abuse laws).

Whereas Chapter 1 was devoted to definitional issues and epidemiological findings with respect to TBI, this chapter will present information relative to the neurological foundations of TBI. Although a comprehensive review of brain development is beyond the scope of this volume (see e.g., Brodal, 1981; Gaddes, 1985; Hynd & Willis, 1988; Lezak, 1983; Reitan & Wolfson, 1985; Rourke, Bakker, Fisk, & Strang, 1983; Spreen, Tupper, Risser, Tuokko, & Edgell, 1984), a basic introduction to these issues is indispensable to understanding traumatic brain injuries. Thus this chapter will focus on describing basic neuroanatomical information and neurodevelopmental theory.

NEUROLOGICAL FOUNDATIONS

The nervous system is divided into two interrelated systems: the central nervous system and the peripheral nervous system. The peripheral nervous system comprises the cranial nerves, the spinal nerves, and the autonomic nervous system, whereas the brain, brain stem, and spinal cord generally are viewed as the primary components of the central nervous system.

15

The peripheral nervous system is crucial in the efficient functioning of the human body and can be disrupted by a traumatic brain injury, but the central nervous system is more generally involved in most brain injuries and will be the focus of this introductory discussion.

Basic Foundations

The human brain is the central organ of the entire human nervous system. It weighs about 1400 grams and constitutes about 2% of total body weight. It is composed of nerve cell bodies, connecting fibers (i.e., axons and dendrites) and their synapses, and supporting cells. These connections contribute to a rapid transmission of information to and from the brain. It has been estimated that the number of nerve cells in the brain falls in the range of approximately 100 billion (Stevens, 1979). Although the process of myelination (i.e., the development of a fatty sheath around the axons and dendrites) contributes to ongoing brain development and growth early in life, the axons and dendrites in a mature nervous system do not multiply in any way. When a nerve cell is damaged, as can be the case in a traumatic brain injury, it may cease to function or its functioning may be altered. When this occurs, brain regions associated with these fibers also may be disrupted, possibly leading to behavioral disruption as well. Furthermore, these cell bodies are oxygen dependent and nourished via a rich venous system. Disturbance of this flow of oxygen via the blood can also cause brain injury. This might be seen in the case of a drowning or a near-drowning event.

As can be seen in Figure 2.1, the brain is an organ that is convoluted in design, with many sulci (the deep furrows) and gyri (raised surfaces). In fact, this design has contributed to the fact that nearly two thirds of the cortex is not visible. It is unclear why this is the case, but it has been speculated that this design serves a survival function in that the majority of the brain is less vulnerable to external trauma. This design also has served to reduce the size of the human head (Gaddes, 1985).

Cerebral Hemispheres

The brain comprises two large cerebral hemispheres, the cerebellum and the brain stem. The left and right hemispheres are the largest parts of the brain and are responsible for higher order cognitive processes (e.g., language, memory, abstract thinking). Although each hemisphere is primarily specialized for specific functions (the left hemisphere tends to be more specialized for language-related functions whereas the right hemisphere tends to be more specialized for visual-perceptual functions), it is important to note that the hemispheres are in constant communication with each other, largely by a bundle of connection fibers called the corpus callosum.

Each hemisphere is further divided into four lobes: occipital, parietal, temporal, and frontal. Two primary sulci provide general divisions for these lobes. The central sulcus provides a general dividing line between the frontal lobe and the parietal lobe. On the anterior side of the central sulcus is the primary motor cortex, which is primarily responsible for motor movements. The left motor cortex is largely responsible for coordinating movements on the right side of the body; the opposite is true for the right motor cortex. On the posterior side of the central sulcus is the primary sensory cortex, which is responsible for tactile sensations. Similar to the motor strip, these right and left cortical regions mediate somatosensory functions on the opposite sides of the body. Taken together, these two cortical regions are referred to as the sensorimotor cortex (Calanchini & Trout, 1971). The second sulcus is the lateral fissure, which divides the temporal lobes and the other lobules. The lobes and the dividing sulci can be seen in Figure 2.1.

Anteriorly, the frontal lobe is the most highly developed part of the brain. In addition to being largely responsible for primary motor movements and motor output, it has been deemed important for organization, planning, evaluation, and the modulation of behavior. In general, the location of the frontal lobes makes them vulnerable to a variety of pedestrian and motor vehicle-related accidents. Immediately posterior to the frontal lobes are the parietal lobes. The parietal lobes have been deemed responsible for processing primary sensory information and mediating selected language and visual-perceptual functions. The temporal lobes are located laterally in the hemispheres, and similar to the frontal lobes, their location contributes to an increased vulnerability to trauma. The temporal lobes house the primary auditory cortex and generally serve to mediate language and selected memory functions. At the most posterior pole are the occipital lobes. The occipital lobes house the primary and secondary visual cortex and mediate functions related to visual perception.

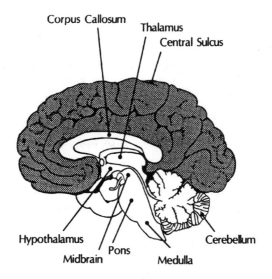

Figure 2.1. The First Functional Unit of the Brain Containing the Brain Stem and Associated Structures.

Brain Stem

In addition to the cerebral hemispheres and their lobules, the brain stem also serves to mediate overall functioning. The brain stem connects with the brain at one end and the spinal cord at the other, and comprises all of the ascending (i.e., entering fibers) and descending (i.e., exiting) hemispheric connections. In general, the brain stem tends to be divided into three major regions: the hindbrain, midbrain, and forebrain. These regions and some of their associated structures are depicted in Figure 2.1.

The lowest division of the brain stem is the hindbrain. The hindbrain contains the medulla oblongata, the reticular formation, the pons, and sections of the cerebellum. The medulla oblongata is responsible for control of respiration, blood pressure, and heartbeat. Given these basic life functions, an injury to this area of the brain can result in a severe vegetative state or instant death. Furthermore, the medulla represents the level where most of the sensory and motor nerves cross over to the opposite side of the body.

The reticular formation is a highly interconnected network of fibers that project to nearly all major neural tracks. In general, the fibers comprising the reticular formation are responsible for complex postural reflexes and muscle tone. The reticular formation also contains the reticular activating system, which regulates wakefulness and general arousal. A traumatic injury to this region can affect an individual's attention, consciousness, and overall arousal.

The pons and the cerebellum can be found higher in the hindbrain and mediate kinesthetic-based movements and coordination. The cerebellum generally has been associated with the maintenance of muscle tone, coordination of muscle groups, and balance, but it also has been linked to selected aspects of sensory processing, perceptual discrimination, and emotionally-based responses (Watson, 1978). Furthermore, a unilateral cerebellar injury may result in paralysis or hemiparesis on the same side of the body as the injury, unlike the contralateral behavioral manifestations of an injury that occurs on one side of the motor strip.

The midbrain contains major sections of the reticular activating system. It also contains nuclei that are primarily responsible for sensory and motor coordination, and contributes to the merging of basic body reflexes related to visual and auditory stimuli. Injuries to this region can produce motor tremors, motor rigidity, and more specific extraneous movement patterns.

The highest part of the brain stem is the forebrain, which is composed of the diencephalon and the telencephalon. The diencephalon is the level where the nerve fibers associated with vision cross, thus contributing to the contralateral cortical representation of the visual fields. Within the diencephalon are two major structures that are important to human functioning: the thalamus and the hypothalamus.

The thalamus contains 11 specific nuclei and reportedly is asymmetric in its organization, much in the same way that the cerebral hemispheres are specialized for specific functions (i.e., the left thalamus is involved in verbal activity whereas the right thalamus is involved in nonverbal activities). Although generally viewed as a major sensory relay station between cortical and subcortical regions (Brodal, 1981), it also has been implicated in regulating cortical activities, focusing and shifting attention, memory retrieval, and mediating selected aspects of emotional functioning.

The hypothalamus is one of the major components of the autonomic nervous system. It has been implicated in appetite, sexual drive, arousal, thirst, and protective functions involving fear and rage. A traumatic brain injury disrupting the hypothalamus can lead to weight problems, particularly obesity, problems with temperature control, fluctuations in mood, and changes in sexual drive.

The telencephalon is the most highly developed region of the forebrain. In addition to giving rise to the two cerebral hemispheres, it contains a number of important subcortical structures. One of these structures is the corpus striatum, or basal ganglia. The basal ganglia represent a group of nuclei that are important for voluntary and involuntary motor movements. An injury to these ganglia can result in motor movement disorders. The internal capsule, a bundled tract of motor fibers, runs through the telencephalon. Another major structure within this region is the amygdala. The amygdala has been associated with the sense of smell as well as visceral behaviors such as salivating, gagging, chewing, and fear.

Summary

This section has served as a brief introduction to the complexities of the human brain. In addition to these basic foundations, it is important to realize that there are many other aspects to brain-behavior relationships that have not been mentioned. For example, the brain is contained in the cranial vault, or skull, which serves as a protective container for the brain tissue. Within the vault, also surrounding the brain, are three membranes that provide further protection of the brain. These layers, or meninges, include the dura mater, the arachnoid, and the pia mater. The meninges are frequently damaged in traumatic brain injuries, which can lead to a variety of medical complications (e.g., epidural hematoma, subdural hematoma, intracranial pressure) that in turn may affect neurobehavioral functioning. Furthermore, this information must be organized within a neurodevelopmental framework for understanding a particular traumatic brain injury in a child at a specific developmental epoch.

NEURODEVELOPMENTAL THEORY

Perhaps one of the most widely accepted and applied neurodevelopmental theories is that asserted by Luria (1966). Luria's theory is founded upon several major concepts, including functional systems, functional units, and cortical zones.

According to Luria (1966), a functional system involves the integrated participation of a number of cortical regions. Consequently, a complex cognitive function, such as reading, could be impaired secondary to damage to any one of a variety of neuroanatomical substrates that make up this functional system. Disruption of this functional system may implicate other cognitive processes as well. This conceptualization of a functional system has allowed for the use of syndrome analysis in systematically reviewing clinical case materials. In addition, this conceptualization paved the way for rehabilitation efforts directed at remediating deficits and/or developing compensatory strategies for regaining a lost function. This conceptualization has established a foundation for many of the rehabilitative efforts with children and adolescents with traumatic brain injury.

Luria (1966) proposed that three functional units of the brain encompassed all functional systems. These units are hierarchically organized and functionally integrated in the planning and execution of cognitive functions. The *first functional unit* is located in subcortical brain regions (i.e., upper and lower parts of the brain stem), and is concerned largely with arousal, wakefulness, and alertness. Impairment in this functional unit can disrupt various components of attention and subsequently interfere with learning and adaptive functioning. Figure 2.1 shows the first functional unit containing the brain stem and some of its associated structures.

The second and third units generally comprise the cortex, with the former encompassing the temporal, parietal, and occipital lobes, and the latter the frontal lobes. The *second functional unit* is responsible for receiving, analyzing, and storing information. Luria (1966) noted that the *third functional unit* contributed to the programming, regulation, and verification of activity. The second and third units are intimately connected to the subcortical structures and are hierarchical in their respective organization. Each of the cortical units contains primary, secondary, and tertiary zones. The second and third units of the brain and their accompanying cortical regions are illustrated in Figure 2.2.

Within the second unit, *primary zones* are modality specific in their functioning. Specific regions within the temporal, parietal, and occipital lobes exclusively process auditory, somatosensory, and visual stimuli, respectively. The primary zones are capable of receiving information from, and sending information to, the periphery. The *secondary zones* of this functional unit, or association regions, process incoming sensory information and relay it to the tertiary regions. Involvement of primary and/or

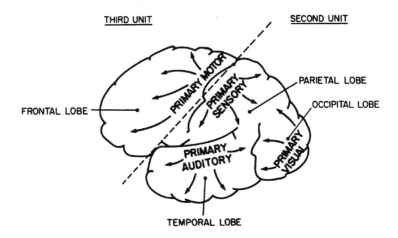

Figure 2.2. The Second and Third Functional Units of the Brain Showing the Four Lobes, Primary Cortical Zones, and the General Sequence of Cortical Maturation.

secondary regions produces behavioral manifestations that are unimodal in appearance. The *tertiary zones* are responsible for the integration of multimodal information and thus higher order, more complex cognitive processes (e.g., reading). Damage involving tertiary regions can contribute to difficulties synthesizing information in an efficient manner (Luria, 1966).

Primary and secondary zones of the third functional unit are responsible for motor movement and organized motor activity, respectively. The tertiary zones have been associated with the planning and execution of goal-directed behaviors. Damage to these regions can result in motor planning and execution deficits. Given their intimate afferent connections with subcortical structures and their involvement in attentional and behavioral modulation, Luria (1966) considered the tertiary, or prefrontal, regions to orchestrate some of the most complex human processes (e.g., problem solving, abstract conceptualization).

Ontogenetically, there is an implicit theory of sequential neurological development that embraces Luria's thinking. This sequence of cortical maturation is shown in Figure 2.2. This sequence of development is dependent upon the physiological and accompanying functional changes that occur with the maturation of various neural substrates. The arousal

unit, largely involving the reticular activating system, generally is operative at birth and is believed to be fully functional by approximately one
year of age. Similarly, the three primary sensory zones and the primary
motor area of the cerebral cortex are intact at birth, with motor development
maturing slightly earlier than sensory functions (Rhawn, 1982).

The secondary cortical regions are the next to develop, and although
beginning to evolve from birth, they are believed to be dominant by about
age 2. The development of skills associated with secondary regions occurs
through about age 5. During this time, the secondary cortical areas are
the major sites of learning, and damage to these regions may affect how
a child learns information and set the stage for later learning differences
or difficulties.

Development of these regions is followed by maturity of the tertiary
areas of the second functional unit. The integrative, polymodal functions
associated with the tertiary temporal-parietal-occipital regions form the
foundation for the acquisition of most formal academic skills, such as
reading and mathematics (Shurtleff, Abbott, Townes, & Berninger, 1990).
Anomalies in these regions have been linked to higher order cognitive
deficits.

The final area to develop is the tertiary region of the frontal lobes.
Injuries to the prefrontal regions have been associated with deficits in attention, abstraction, cognitive flexibility, planning, sequential processing, self-
evaluation and monitoring of performance, and visual organization (Stuss
& Benson, 1986). In fact, lesions to these areas can remain "silent" until
challenged later or until age-appropriate social, behavioral, and cognitive
demands are required of the child (Rourke et al., 1983). This is especially
pertinent to the later development of a young child who receives a traumatic brain injury to this region. If these skills and abilities are not tapped
in a subsequent assessment, they may be missed, and the child may be viewed
as having incurred no cognitive residuals from the injury. This, in turn,
may pave the way for damaging misinterpretations to occur with respect
to a child's functioning, particularly as the maturation process ensues.

SUMMARY

As can be seen from the preceding discussion, understanding basic neurological foundations and having a working knowledge of neurodevelop-

mental theory are extremely important with respect to providing clearer interpretive conceptualizations as well as developing a foundation for prognostic and prescriptive endeavors for children and adolescents sustaining a traumatic brain injury. Luria's (1966) concept of a functional system also has allowed for flexibility in how to intervene with an individual following a traumatic brain injury, particularly with respect to cognitive and/or physical retraining. His model offers a comprehensive framework for developmental neuropsychological assessment and subsequent monitoring. Another crucial area to understanding a traumatic brain injury, however, is the neuropathological mechanism by which a specific type of traumatic brain injury was sustained. Some of these issues will be examined in the next chapter.

Part II

Neuropathological Mechanisms and Outcomes

3

NEUROPATHOLOGICAL MECHANISMS AND TYPES OF INJURIES

In this chapter, we will describe the basic neuropathological mechanisms that lead to different types of brain injury. These mechanisms are noteworthy given the effort nature has devoted to protecting the brain (e.g., convolutions, skull). Understanding the different types of injuries and their associated mechanisms can help the child practitioner begin to establish assessment strategies and associated hypotheses with respect to outcome possibilities. In addition, there are a number of secondary medical effects that can be seen with the different types of traumatic brain injuries; these will be mentioned briefly for the purpose of assessing their potential impact upon an individual's acute neurobehavioral status as well as ultimate recovery of function.

NEUROPATHOLOGICAL MECHANISMS

The mechanisms involved in a traumatic brain injury primarily result from three basic physical forces: tension (the tearing apart of tissues), compression (the pushing together of brain tissue), and shearing (the sliding of one portion of tissue over another). These physical forces combine to describe injuries from acceleration-dependent (acceleration, deceleration, rotation) and nonacceleration-dependent factors (e.g., crushing injuries). The latter injuries are relatively rare, and as much of the physical energy is evenly distributed, these injuries typically cause skull fractures, but relatively little brain damage. In such cases, the amount of brain damage is largely dependent upon the degree of skull deformation. Given the relative rarity of these types of injuries, acceleration-dependent injuries will be the primary focus of this discussion.

Acceleration-Dependent Injuries

Over 50 years ago, Denny-Brown and Russell (1941) demonstrated that a moderate blow to a movable head could produce severe brain damage, but a blow with 20 times the strength could be sustained by a rigidly fixed head with relatively little brain damage being incurred. Although clinical situations involving a rigidly fixed head are infrequent (i.e., nonacceleration-dependent factors), acceleration forces typically have been viewed as the dominant factors involved in traumatic brain injuries, particularly closed head injuries (Pang, 1985). Examples of this type of injury would be an individual receiving a blow to the head from a punch, baseball, or rock.

Acceleration injuries occur when the slower moving brain tissue is damaged or rendered dysfunctional by a sudden external force. The brain tissue is of a different density than bone, and consequently accelerates at a slower rate than bone. As the external force or object hits the head, the skull moves in a direction opposite the impact whereas the brain tissue initially moves in the direction of the impact and then follows the direction of the skull.

In contrast to pure accelerating forces, where an object strikes a stationary head, deceleration forces occur when the moving head strikes a stationary object. In these instances, such as in motor vehicle accidents, the head is suddenly stopped with resultant damage possibly occurring at the impact site (i.e., coup), and also at the opposite site (i.e., contrecoup).

Rotational injuries occur as a result of hyperflexion, hyperextension, lateral flexion, and turning movements of the head on the neck and brain stem. These rotational, or torquing, forces can produce shearing and tearing of cerebral tissue, with some investigators attributing most contrecoup injuries to these forces (Ommaya, Grubbs, & Naumann, 1971). All of these mechanisms can result in the rupturing of superficial and deep blood vessels, and the subsequent development of different kinds of hemorrhages.

Acceleration-dependent forces also may be subdivided into translational and angular types. If the resultant vector of an external force passes through the center of gravity of the body, the body assumes translational, or linear, acceleration along the direction of the force. In contrast, if the

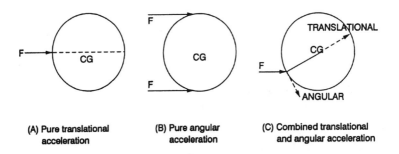

(A) Pure translational acceleration

(B) Pure angular acceleration

(C) Combined translational and angular acceleration

Figure 3.1. The Effects of Different Forces Acting on a Rigid Spherical Body

A. A single force (F) passing through the center of gravity (CG) of the body produces pure translational acceleration.
B. Pure angular acceleration results from two simultaneous opposing forces of equal magnitude directed at opposite sides of CG.
C. A single force not passing through the CG will produce combined translational and angular motions with both types of acceleration.
SOURCE: Pang (1985). Reprinted with permission.

external force does not create a vector that passes through the center of gravity of a body, then angular acceleration occurs, and the body rotates around its own center of gravity. Pure angular acceleration occurs only when the body is acted on by two opposing forces of equal magnitude on opposite sides of the center of gravity. In general, most traumatic brain injuries are a combination of translational and angular forces, and more rarely reflect one type or the other. Also, because the head is attached to the spinal cord via the brain stem, some degree of rotation always tends to occur regardless of the direction of the impact (Pang, 1985). These types of acceleration forces can be seen in Figure 3.1.

Another factor seen with acceleration-dependent injuries is the effect of positive and negative pressure zones. Lindenberg and Freytag (1960) attributed brain contusions, or the coup injuries, to the positive pressure zone that is created immediately beneath the impact site where the brain moves toward the skull, and the contrecoup injuries to the negative pressure zone directly opposite the site of impact. According to the cavitation theory, contrecoup injuries actually can be more frequent and more pronounced in terms of involved brain regions and severity than the coup injury. This is suspected due to the tearing and shearing of fibers caused by the negative pressure (Gilroy & Meyer, 1979; Spatz, 1950). The cavitation theory satisfactorily explains many of the lesions typically seen in traumatic brain injuries; however, it does not account for other neuroanatomical lesions that can be seen in deeper brain structures (e.g., hypothalamus) (Pang, 1985).

TYPES OF TRAUMATIC
BRAIN INJURIES

Prior to discussing the different types of brain injuries that might be seen, it is important to note that a trauma to the head does not always lead to a brain injury (Boll, 1983). From a TBI perspective, to be of clinical significance to the pediatric neurologist, child psychologist, or other child practitioner, a head trauma must be sufficient to produce a disruption of the central nervous system. Several types of brain injuries, with two broad classes, are generally accepted: penetrating wounds/injuries and nonpenetrating injuries. Other investigators suggest a third category, skull fractures (Gilroy & Meyer, 1979), but this will be subsumed under the two broad classes.

Penetrating Head Injuries

Penetrating head injuries occur when an external object strikes the head, typically via acceleration-dependent forces, with sufficient strength to cause a depressed skull fracture, and skull fragments either tear the dura or cause a brain laceration. About 30% of all skull fractures reportedly are of a depressed nature (Reitan & Wolfson, 1985), with compound fractures being present in about 20% of children with severe head trauma (Burkinshaw, 1960).

A second kind of penetrating head injury occurs when a missile penetrates the skull. Such a penetration can lead to the missile being lodged in the brain tissue or passing through it. Some individuals may show an immediate loss of consciousness; others may not lose consciousness at the time of injury, but gradually progress into a coma state over several hours. If the injury is severe enough, increased intracranial pressure and decreased blood pressure may be seen, and in turn, may create a medical emergency. Problems associated with brain stem functions also can be observed (e.g., arousal).

In penetrating brain injuries, both focal and diffuse effects can be observed. Tearing of the dura and subsequent damage to the underlying vasculature of the dura and meninges along with focal contusions can be observed in such cases. Furthermore, the depressed skull fragments can cause tearing of the brain tissue directly underlying the depression (Dacey, Alves, Rimel, Winn, & Jane, 1986; Menkes & Batzdorf, 1985; Shapiro, 1987). Diffuse effects, such as stretching and shearing of the brain tissue, as well as contrecoup contusions also may occur with penetrating types of brain injuries (Fennell & Mickle, 1992) although these consequences are less likely. Brain contusions (bruising) most often can be seen in depressed skull fractures (Shapiro, 1987). Here, loss of consciousness does not occur fre- quently, but the risk of seizures is higher.

Nonpenetrating Head Injuries

In contrast to the penetrating injuries, nonpenetrating head injuries do not involve any actual penetration of foreign material into the brain. These injuries can occur when the trauma to the head does not produce a skull fracture, or the trauma generates a nondepressed, or linear, skull fracture. This type of involvement includes closed head injuries and concussions, and in general accounts for over 90% of major pediatric head injuries (Menkes, 1985).

Although a head injury can occur at any time in life, infants and young children are at particular risk for nonpenetrating closed head injuries, largely because of specific skull-brain interface factors. For example, at birth there are six spaces, or fontanelles, between the neonatal skull bones. These remain unfused to accommodate the increasing size of the brain. Five of these fontanelles fuse by the age of 6 weeks, but the most anterior one does not fuse until somewhere between the ages of 9 to 16 months. As one might suspect, the infant brain is particularly susceptible to damage during this period, although the flexibility of the immature skull enables it to absorb a greater degree of deformation before fracturing (Menkes, 1985). This absorption factor, however, also has the potential to contribute to increased generalized shearing damage to the brain (Courville, 1965).

The interface between the skull and the brain also affects the different kinds of brain damage that can be seen. The brain tends to be more tightly packed in the posterior regions of the brain and more loosely packed in anterior regions, and because the brain is more tightly packed in posterior regions, the internal surface of the skull tends to be smoother, whereas an increased number of bony protuberances can be found in the anterior regions.

Consequently, the frontal and temporal lobes, particularly anterior temporal regions, are the cortical areas most likely to be damaged, regardless of the site or direction of the initial impact. Thus frontotemporal lacerations and contusions are frequently seen in all types of brain injuries, particularly nonpenetrating head injuries (Bigler, 1990). These injuries, in turn, can result in memory disorders, executive functioning deficits, and a variety of emotional changes (Levin et al., 1982; Salazar et al., 1986).

Another primary attribute of head injuries of all types is diffuse axonal injuries. Neuropathological data suggest that the predominant impact of traumatic brain injury is of a diffuse, nonspecific nature (Adams, Graham, & Gennarelli, 1985; Jennett, 1986). This is especially evident in cases of closed head injury. Even when focal deficits are evidenced, they typically are present in the face of more diffuse findings as well. These diffuse findings have been related to the effects of neuronal shearing and tearing (Auerbach, 1986). The diffuse damage that occurs results from the twisting, tearing, or breaking of the axonal fibers, damage to the connective supporting cells of the brain, or neuronal degeneration. These processes are collectively referred to as diffuse axonal injury. Diffuse axonal injury can occur anywhere in the brain, but typically occurs in the brain stem, deep white-matter structures, and in the frontal and temporal regions. These processes can be seen in Figure 3.2.

SECONDARY MEDICAL COMPLICATIONS

A number of secondary medical complications can arise following a traumatic brain injury. Many of these concerns will be addressed prior to a child or adolescent leaving the hospital or rehabilitation setting, but it is important for the child practitioner to be aware of these complications as they may impact upon an individual's physical, neurocognitive, and general adaptive functioning. These include hypoxia/ischemia, cerebral edema, hemorrhage, cerebral atrophy and ventricular enlargement, and posttraumatic epilepsy.

Hypoxia/Ischemia

In addition to the neuronal shearing and tearing effects that can be seen with diffuse axonal injury, neuronal damage also can occur via obstructed blood flow (ischemia) and/or poorly oxygenated blood (hypoxia). Frequent-

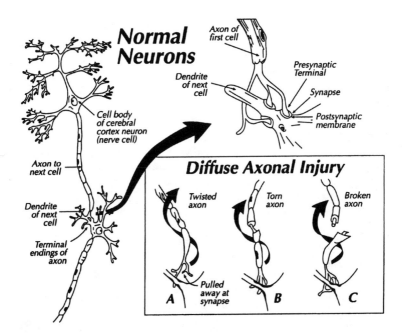

Figure 3.2. A Schematic Illustrating Normal Neurons and the Different
Mechanisms by Which Diffuse Axonal Injury to the Neuron Can Occur.
SOURCE: Adapted from Bigler (1990). Reprinted with permission.

ly, a loss of blood pressure to the brain can be seen, perhaps secondary to
a significant loss of blood. When pressure falls to a certain critical point,
ischemic hypoxia can occur. This process in turn can contribute to brain
tissue damage or destruction, particularly in the small vessels of the brain.
In addition to the diffuse effects that can be seen with ischemic hypoxia,
there are some data suggesting that anoxic-type damage tends to disrupt
the hippocampus, which can lead to memory deficits.

Cerebral Edema

Cerebral edema, or brain swelling, is the most common secondary effect
of traumatic brain injury. It can create focal findings, such as with a lateralized contusion, or it can produce more generalized findings (Yoshino,
Yamaki, Higuchi, Horikawa, & Hirakawa, 1985). Prolonged cerebral edema

can compress blood vessels feeding the brain and lead to an infarction. It also can create brain cell and/or axonal dysfunction or damage (Ito, Tomita, Yamazaki, Takada, & Inaba, 1986).

Children appear to be at a greater risk than adults for developing diffuse cerebral swelling following a traumatic brain injury. Shapiro (1987) estimated that about 30% of conscious head-injured children and about 40% of comatose children show diffuse cerebral edema on computed axial tomography (CT scan). With the possibility of tissue damage and destruction, concomitant neuropsychological sequelae typically can be seen.

Hemorrhage

Hemorrhages are bleeds that can occur in nearly any place in the brain. An extradural hematoma is a collection of blood between the skull and the dura that develops at the site of the trauma; it occurs in about 1% of children hospitalized for traumatic brain injury and typically is unilateral in its appearance. The severity of symptoms is associated in part with the size of the hematoma and the speed of its evolution. In children, there typically is a period of disorientation or loss of consciousness, but neurologic signs can appear and a progressive loss of consciousness can ensue minutes to days after the evolution of the hematoma (Kissock et al., 1960; Mealey, 1968). In general, the younger the child, the longer the latency. Seizures can occur, but are rare (Hendrick, Harwood-Nash, & Hudson, 1963). Mealey (1968) also noted that in nearly 40% of children with extradural hematoma, a skull fracture was not detectable by radiologic examination.

A subdural hematoma is a localized collection of blood between the dura and the cerebral mantle and typically has neurosurgical implications due to increased intracranial pressure. It typically is unilateral in its appearance (Menkes, 1985), although it can be bilateral, and is responsible for death and physical injury in a significant number of battered or shaken babies (Caffey, 1974).

In this connection, it is important to reiterate that a hematoma may form at the time of the injury, or sometime thereafter, so it might not be an immediate complication from a traumatic brain injury (Bucci, Phillips, & McGillicuddy, 1986; Soloniuk, Pitts, Lovely, & Bartkowski, 1986). The presence of any type of hematoma, regardless of location, may exacerbate underlying cerebral dysfunction or damage and might be related to increased risk for neurocognitive deficits (Cullum & Bigler, 1986).

Cerebral Atrophy and Ventricular Enlargement

Traumatic brain injury also can cause cerebral atrophy, which typically corresponds to enlargement of the ventricular system via hydrocephalus (Cullum & Bigler, 1986; Levin, Meyers, Grossman, & Sarwar, 1981; Lipper et al., 1985). Cullum and Bigler (1986) noted that this atrophy tends to be evidenced more in the frontal and temporal regions, although it also can present in a diffuse fashion, with the greatest atrophy being associated with areas of contusion and/or prior hematoma. White-matter degeneration also has been described in the pediatric age group (Graham, Adams, & Gennarelli, 1987) and typically results from retraction of axonal pathways following injury. In traumatic brain injury, however, it has been suggested by neuroimaging procedures that changes in ventricular size may be more sensitive to structural deficits than the actual presence of cortical atrophy.

Posttraumatic Epilepsy

Seizures associated with a traumatic brain injury have been classified by their time of onset following an injury. Immediate types of seizures occur within a few seconds of the head trauma. Menkes (1985) suspects that these types of seizures are the result of direct mechanical stimulation of brain tissue having a low seizure threshold. Early types of seizures typically appear during the first 24 to 48 hours following a brain injury. In general, these are due to cerebral edema, intracranial hemorrhage, contusion, laceration, or actual tissue necrosis.

Children are more prone to develop seizures in the immediate and early postinjury period than adults, although the overall incidence of early posttraumatic seizures is about 7% (Jennett, 1975). Jennett (1975) noted that children were more likely than adults to experience early posttraumatic seizures after minor head trauma, but do not appear to be at any greater risk to develop posttraumatic epilepsy later (Annegers et al., 1980). Depressed skull fractures tend to occur in many of these children (Hendrick et al., 1963). Late posttraumatic seizures tend to emerge within 2 years following the injury, with about 50% of these occurring within the first year. These seizures typically have their origin in cerebromeningeal scarring (Grand, 1974).

Furthermore, there is a 5% to 10% incidence of posttraumatic epilepsy in children who experienced a loss of consciousness for at least one hour following their traumatic brain injury, compared to a 2% occurrence when there was not a significant loss of consciousness. This incidence rate increased to 30% when a brain laceration was sustained and doubled when the child experienced a posttraumatic amnesia of more than 24 hours.

The topography of these seizures can take any form, but as a general rule, the topography is not manifested in absence form. It has been estimated that these seizures become less frequent after the third year following the injury in about 20% to 50% of patients, but that the individual remains prone to a seizure disorder (Jennett, 1975). Finally, it also must be remembered that many of the anticonvulsant medications also maintain their own liabilities with respect to their impact on neurocognitive functioning (e.g., phenytoin and phenobarbital both can cause or contribute to selective deficits on neuropsychological testing).

SUMMARY

In this chapter, we have attempted to provide a brief overview of the multitude of factors that can evolve as the result of a traumatic brain injury. For the child clinician, understanding the different neuropathological mechanisms involved in a traumatic brain injury, the types of head injury that can arise, and the subsequent medical complications that can be present is crucial to planning assessment, diagnostic, and prognostic venues for an individual child or adolescent. Understanding these processes, along with the neurological foundations of traumatic brain injury, sets the stage for conceptualizing the plethora of neurobehavioral and psychosocial outcomes that can be found in children and adolescents suffering such trauma.

4

NEUROCOGNITIVE AND PSYCHOSOCIAL OUTCOMES

With a basic understanding of the neuropathological mechanisms and the different types of traumatic head injuries that can occur, we now move into a discussion of outcomes. In general, the behavioral sequelae of head trauma have been reported as less severe in children than in adults (Heiskanen & Sipponen, 1970), although this has been seriously challenged in recent years (Fletcher, Miner, & Ewing-Cobbs, 1987). As might be expected from such a heterogeneous group of patients, the range of neurocognitive and psychosocial outcomes can be highly varied. In addition, there may be any number of medical outcomes, some of which were described in the preceding chapter, that continue to interfere with the accurate assessment of an individual's functioning (e.g., posttraumatic seizures, spasticity, ataxia). For most pediatric patients, outcome continues to be defined largely by school attendance, school performance, neuropsychological functioning, and parent/teacher reports of cognitive and emotional symptoms. In this chapter, we focus on the neurocognitive and psychosocial outcomes that have been reported in children and adolescents who have sustained a traumatic brain injury.

NEUROCOGNITIVE OUTCOMES
IN PENETRATING HEAD INJURIES

When the brain is damaged, deficits stem from injury to those areas of the brain that govern the involved functions. In penetrating head injuries, such as injury sustained from a bullet, discrete brain areas in the path of injury are typically affected with largely predictable deficits. For example, if a bullet passes through the right motor strip, then it is likely that involvement (e.g., paralysis) of structures on the left side of the body will result.

In general, although the incidence of penetrating head injuries is difficult to ascertain, it has been estimated that only about 2% to 5% of all head injuries brought to medical attention are penetrating types of injuries (Kampen & Grafman, 1989), and this figure is lower for children and adolescents. This speculation is bolstered when one takes into account that the major penetrating head injuries typically occur as a result of military combat, suicide attempts, crime, or miscellaneous accidents during work or leisure activities.

The amount and kind of tissue damage incurred from a penetrating head injury depend on a number of factors, including the type of object, the brain location of entry, and the velocity of the object. For example, studies investigating the effects of high-velocity missile injuries have evidenced microscopic changes in brain regions far from the actual missile track, whereas the changes incurred from low-velocity objects (e.g., a knife) typically show focal damage. Furthermore, a penetrating object can enter the brain at any particular point and then perform a number of actions. It can come to rest along the original missile trajectory, ricochet within the skull cavity, break apart and leave shrapnel and bone fragments scattered along the path and in adjacent and distal brain regions, or exit the skull. The penetrating injury also can produce hemorrhaging (Kaufman, Makela, Lee, Haid, & Gildenberg, 1986), although contrecoup injuries are rarely observed.

Given the relatively high variability in these types of injuries, systematic neurobehavioral studies are few. A recent study of six patients (Kampen & Grafman, 1989), four adults and two children with penetrating wounds from gunshots, showed focal deficits at one year postinjury (e.g., the patients with left hemisphere injuries exhibited greater verbal difficulties) as opposed to any generalized lowering of neurocognitive abilities. In addition, however, all of the patients evidenced some form of memory dysfunction.

In summary, deficits from a penetrating head injury should in large part directly relate to the areas of the brain that were damaged by the object. Other regions of the brain also may be affected, however, depending on the actions of the object and the response to the object by the brain. Nonetheless, if a child practitioner can recognize the entry point of an object, and perhaps its exit point, initial functional hypotheses can be established based on what is known about brain-behavior relationships in childhood.

NEUROCOGNITIVE OUTCOMES
IN NONPENETRATING HEAD INJURIES

Nonpenetrating head injuries can result in more diffuse brain damage. Although primary damage can occur to structures at the point of impact, damage also may occur at the point opposite the impact point (i.e., contrecoup injury) when the brain is pushed against the interior of the skull. Secondary injury results from processes of vasodilation, edema, and increased intracranial pressure that occur as a result of the primary injury. For example, if the right-sided motor strip is the point of impact, then left-sided motor involvement (e.g., hemiparesis) may occur; however, a right-sided motor problem may arise as a consequence of the contrecoup injury from the more generalized secondary injury.

In its least severe form, a nonpenetrating, or closed head injury, can produce a concussion. A concussion is a brief alteration in or loss of consciousness. This is usually followed by a period of confusion, disorientation, and other neurological signs such as bradycardia, lowering of the blood pressure, and amnesia (Gennarelli, 1986). In children, these symptoms can be delayed for minutes or hours after a traumatic head injury, with full recovery typically occurring within 24 hours (Shapiro, 1987). Postconcussion syndrome occurring during childhood includes headaches, irritability, physical lethargy, emotional lability, memory disruption, and associated academic performance problems (Casey, Ludwig, & McCormick, 1986; Lanser, Jennekens-Schinkel, & Peters, 1988; Levin, Magnusson, Rafto, & Zimmerman, 1989).

In addition to the range of symptoms that can be seen in childhood postconcussion syndrome, a variety of other neurocognitive outcomes have been advanced with respect to children and adolescents with nonpenetrating types of brain injuries. These outcomes have been reviewed in detail, particularly for the closed head injury literature, and span intellectual, motor, attention, language, visual perceptual, memory, and academic functional domains (Ewing-Cobbs & Fletcher, in press; Fennell & Mickle, 1992). Selected findings in each of these domains will be highlighted here.

Intellectual Performance

A review of numerous studies exploring the possibility of a decline in the level of intellectual performance following a traumatic brain injury reveals a clear trend in that direction. Klonoff, Low, and Clark (1977) showed that initial level of intellectual function estimates on a large group of children and adolescents with TBI were significantly below a matched group of normal controls. Levin and Eisenberg (1979a) reported a low average level of intellectual functioning for children who were comatose for at least 24 hours. For severely involved children (i.e., GCS ≤ 7 or a PTA ≥ 7 days), scores on the Wechsler Intelligence Scale for Children—Revised typically have evidenced lower Performance IQs as compared to Verbal IQs (Chadwick et al., 1981; Levin & Eisenberg, 1979a; Winogron, Knights, & Bawden, 1984). It has been suspected that this pattern of results likely is due to the dependence of many of the verbal subtests on old learning, with the exception of Arithmetic and Digit Span, whereas subtests from the performance scale are more dependent upon speeded accuracy, problem solving, and novel learning (Boll, 1983).

It is unlikely that IQ scores return to preinjury levels for severely brain-injured children, with evidence indicating that only a partial recovery of intellectual abilities may be possible (Levin & Eisenberg, 1979b; Mayes, Pelco, & Campbell, 1989; Richardson, 1963). This has been buttressed by studies showing persistent IQ deficits at 1 year (Berger-Gross & Shackelford, 1985; Chadwick et al., 1981), 2.5 years (Chadwick et al., 1981), 3 years (Filley, Cranberg, Alexander, & Hart, 1987), 4 years (Mahoney et al., 1983), and 5 years (Klonoff et al., 1977) postinjury. Although these findings appear to be related directly to the severity of the head injury, they seem to be robust for younger as well as older children.

Motor/Visual-Motor Functions

As Shapiro (1987) noted, the assessment of motor functions following a traumatic brain injury typically has been conducted as part of the neurological examination. Focal signs of motor dysfunction, such as hemiparesis, facial weakness, and problems with balance and gait, typically have been described. Several studies, however, have attempted to document motor functioning in a more explicit fashion.

Levin et al. (1982) described motor slowing during the immediate time period following a mild, moderate, or severe head injury, although the severity of the injury begins to exert a significant influence on the chronicity of these deficits. Gulbrandsen (1984) reported that mildly head-injured children did not differ from normal controls on simple motor speed at 6 months postinjury. For a severely injured group, however, simple and complex motor speed deficits have been documented, with these deficits persisting through 1-year (Bawden, Knights, & Winogron, 1985; Chadwick et al., 1981; Winogron et al., 1984) and 2-year follow-up points (Klonoff et al., 1977).

Visual-motor deficits also have been reported, particularly in copying and construction abilities (Bawden et al., 1985; Chadwick et al., 1981; Klonoff et al., 1977; Levin & Eisenberg, 1979a, 1979b). In fact, Chadwick et al. (1981) uncovered these types of problems regardless of which hemisphere was involved.

Attention

Attentional problems for children and adolescents following a traumatic brain injury have been described across several studies, with these observations again surfacing largely for the more severely injured group (Black, Jeffries, Blumer, Wellner, & Walker, 1969; Bruce, Schut, Bruno, Wood, & Sutton, 1978). Hyperactivity and poor attention have been reported by parents at follow-up intervals (Brink, Hale, Woo-Sam, & Nickel, 1970), with some evidence suggesting that these deficits can persist in a younger age group for up to 5 years postinjury (Klonoff et al., 1977). Deficits in concentration and speeded performance have been documented through 1 year postinjury for traumatic-brain-injured children at all levels of severity (Bawden et al., 1985; Winogron et al., 1984), although these findings have not been universally supported (Chadwick et al., 1981). Obviously, how attention and its various components are operationally defined and measured potentially influence these types of findings, and these issues continue to require refinement for study in TBI populations (Fennell & Mickle, 1992).

Language

In general, the incidence of speech and language deficits following a traumatic brain injury increases proportionately with the degree of severity (Levin & Eisenberg, 1979a). More pervasive deficits, such as mutism and frank aphasias, can be seen in many children, particularly those with severe head injuries (Ylvisaker, 1986). These types of global deficits tend to occur in younger children (i.e., less than 5 years), although Hecaen (1976) noted that these deficits tend to improve over the process of recovery.

More contemporary estimates of aphasic-type disorders secondary to a head injury have ranged from about one third of pediatric closed head injury patients (Kaiser & Pfenninger, 1984) to nearly two thirds of severely brain-injured individuals (Gilchrist & Wilkinson, 1979).

In addition to these global speech/language deficits, specific deficits also have been uncovered. A variety of studies have shown specific deficits following a traumatic brain injury in object naming (Chadwick et al., 1981; Jordon, Ozanne, & Murdoch, 1990; Levin & Eisenberg, 1979a, 1979b), verbal fluency (Chadwick et al., 1981; Slater & Bassett, 1988; Winogron et al., 1984), word and sentence repetition (Levin & Eisenberg, 1979a, 1979b), speech (Filley et al., 1987), and written output (Ewing-Cobbs, Levin, Eisenberg, & Fletcher, 1987). From a developmental perspective, Ewing-Cobbs, Fletcher, Levin, and Landry (1985) speculated that the type of speech/language impairment incurred from a traumatic brain injury is related to the language skills that are in primary ascendancy at the time of the injury.

Memory

Despite the high degree of interaction between memory functions and attentional efficiency, a variety of memory deficits typically can be seen in children and adolescents following a severe traumatic brain injury, particularly in children suffering from closed head injuries (Fennell & Mickle, 1992). Similar to other functional domains, memory deficits secondary to mild and moderate brain injuries are less clear, especially over the long term. Bassett and Slater (1990) showed deficits in immediate and delayed recall of story passages and visual reproductions in their sample of severely involved adolescents; however, these deficits were not manifested in their mildly injured or age-matched normal controls. Similarly, deficits in visual recall (Berger-Gross & Shackelford, 1985; Klonoff et al., 1977; Levin et al., 1988) and spatial memory (Winogron et al., 1984) have been reported in severe TBI groups at 1 year postinjury, but these deficits tended not to be present in milder injuries beyond 6 to 12 months postinjury. A similar trend has been observed for verbally based memory functions (Chadwick et al., 1981; Levin & Eisenberg, 1979a, 1979b; Levin, Eisenberg, Wigg, & Kobayashi, 1982), particularly for verbal retrieval of newly learned materials.

Academic

Surprisingly, relatively few systematic studies have been conducted examining the academic morbidity following a traumatic brain injury. This is surprising given that a child spends nearly the equivalent of a work week in the school setting. One crucial distinction needs to be made with respect to understanding the academic functioning of children and adolescents with a traumatic brain injury. This is the distinction between skill-based deficits and performance-based deficits. Skill-based deficits reflect a lack of knowledge or ability regarding a specific academic domain (i.e., the skills are not present or have deteriorated secondary to a TBI), whereas performance-based deficits reflect the actual execution of skills and abilities that may be present. It is speculated that clinicians should expect to see skill- and perhaps performance-based deficits at younger ages, and performance-based deficiencies at older ages. Although intuitive, this speculation requires further substantiation (Ewing-Cobbs et al., 1985; Rutter, 1981).

To date, academic problems following traumatic brain injury at all severity levels have covered the gamut, although these findings typically have been seen for children and adolescents suffering moderate to severe injuries. In addition to specific problems in reading (Shaffer, Bijur, Chadwick, & Rutter, 1980), writing (Berger-Gross & Shackleford, 1985), and arithmetic (Levin & Benton, 1986), several investigators have documented the increased need for special education programs, failure to return to school, and a tendency to be placed in a lower grade placement upon school reentry (Brink et al., 1970; Flach & Malmros, 1972; Fuld & Fisher, 1977; Heiskanen & Kaste, 1974; Klonoff et al., 1977). For example, Klonoff et al. (1977) demonstrated that over one quarter of their younger sample (i.e., younger than 9 years) had either failed a grade or been placed in a special education class, whereas one fifth of the older group received special education placements. These rates are impressive, particularly in light of the large number of milder injuries represented in this sample.

The variety of deficits that can be manifested in children and adolescents with traumatic brain injury truly is impressive, and their impact undoubtedly affects school performance—even with mild injuries. Difficulties learning new or novel materials, problems with higher order cognition (e.g., generalization, abstraction, organization, planning, strategy generation), slowed information processing, and poor independent work efforts all can impact a child's classroom performance in a negative fashion. These difficulties should be taken into account when evaluating a TBI survivor's return to the formal academic setting.

PSYCHOSOCIAL OUTCOMES IN TRAUMATIC BRAIN INJURIES

From all available evidence to date, it is clear that a traumatic brain injury can be associated with increased vulnerability for social-emotional adjustment difficulties or for the emergence of a psychiatric disorder. For example, Klonoff and Paris (1974) found that for their younger age group (ages 2 to 8 years), denial of the injury and lack of concern for the injury were the most common reactions. For their older group (ages 9 through 15), however, they noted a significant deterioration in self-concept.

Some examinations have suggested that behavior problems may emerge in the initial time period following even a mild head trauma (Casey et al., 1986). In this regard, although studies of children with mild- to-moderate brain injuries have evidenced changes in temperament and other transient behavioral symptoms (e.g., increased irritability) immediately following an injury (Brown, Chadwick, Shaffer, Rutter, & Traub, 1981; Casey et al., 1986), mild head injuries do not appear to be associated with an increased risk for psychiatric disturbance. The same cannot be said with respect to more severe traumatic brain injuries.

Probably one of the best controlled examinations of this topic comes from the prospective studies of head-injured children by Rutter and his colleagues (Brown et al., 1981; Chadwick, Rutter, Brown, Shaffer, & Traub, 1981; Chadwick, Rutter, Shaffer, & Shrout, 1981; Rutter et al., 1980). Children ranging from 5 to 14 years of age who had experienced closed head injuries of sufficient severity to result in posttraumatic amnesia (PTA) of 7 days or more were compared with a group of children having less severe head injuries (PTA less than 7 days, but a duration of at least 1 hour). In addition, these groups were compared with a matched control group of hospital-treated children also suffering severe accidents, but with orthopedic rather than cranial injuries. All children were studied prospectively at 4 months, 1 year, and 2.5 years after their injuries. An important feature of this study was the care taken to determine the children's behavior before their accident. This was done in an unbiased fashion by interviewing parents immediately after their child's injury, but *before* the child's postinjury psychiatric condition could have been known.

The children with severe head injuries did not differ from controls in their preinjury behavior, but they showed more than double the rate of psychiatric disorder at 4 months postinjury, and at each subsequent follow-up point. This was true even when children who had psychiatric disorders before their accident were eliminated from the study, thereby focusing specifically on the comparative rate of new psychiatric disorders arising over the course of the follow-up period. There was a rather high threshold for an effect, however, because definite cognitive or psychiatric sequelae were found only in head-injured children having a PTA of at least one week.

Whereas persistent psychiatric sequelae were quite common once this range of severity was reached, cognitive impairment lasting for more than 2 years generally required a PTA of at least 3 weeks. Head-injured children tended to show greater impairment on timed visual-spatial and visual-motor tests than on verbal tests, but apart from this, no pattern of cognitive deficits specific to head injury was identified. Likewise, the types of psychiatric disorder among the head-injured children were very similar to those found in controls. The only exception to this was in the case of grossly disinhibited social behavior, which was present only in children with very severe head injuries and may have been linked directly to frontal lobe damage or dysfunction. As can be seen in Figure 4.1, the rate of new psychiatric disorders in the severe head injury group was significantly increased, but the rates in the mildly injured group and the controls were equivocal.

Children with severe head injuries showed an increased risk for psychiatric disorder regardless of the age, sex, or social class of the child—factors that ordinarily show a striking mediating effect in the general population. The risk also was greater among children with histories of preaccident behavior disorders as well as those experiencing various psychosocial adversities within their homes, but the effects were additive rather than interactive. Thus, although psychiatric disorders in childhood have a multifactorial etiology, evidence from this series of studies indicated that severe brain injury can play a major independent role in the development

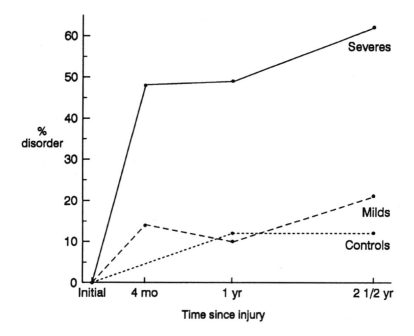

Figure 4.1. Rates of "New" Psychiatric Disorder Following Orthopedic or Head Injuries of Children.
SOURCE: Brown, Chadwick, Shaffer, Rutter, and Traub (1981). Reprinted with permission.

or exacerbation of psychosocial difficulties, whereas mild head injuries do not.

These trends have been uncovered by other investigators as well (Filley et al., 1987; Gulbransen, 1984; Klonoff et al., 1977; Levin et al., 1989; Michaud, Rivara, Jafe, Fay, & Dailey, 1993). In fact, poor social adjustment difficulties from severe head injuries in children have ranged from about 25% at 1 year postinjury (Klonoff et al., 1977), to more than 50% at about 3 (Filley et al., 1987) and 5 years postinjury (Klonoff et al., 1977). More recently, Fletcher, Ewing-Cobbs, Miner, Levin, and Eisenberg (1990) reported that their sample of children with severe head injuries showed significant decline in adaptive behaviors at 1 year postinjury when compared to children with mild traumatic brain injuries. Their severely injured children also were reported to be involved in fewer social and school activities. These findings are illustrated in Figure 4.2. The similarities to the findings by Rutter et al. (1981) are striking and suggest some degree of consistency in the data-based conclusions regarding the psychosocial outcomes of individuals with severe traumatic brain injuries.

FACTORS INFLUENCING OUTCOMES

In addition to rehabilitation efforts, which will be discussed in Chapter 8, there are a variety of factors that influence rate of recovery of functions and ultimate outcome. Many of these factors have been mentioned already, such as types of injuries (penetrating versus nonpenetrating; localized and/or generalized damage), medical complications (brain edema, posttraumatic seizure, intracranial pressure), and injury severity (e.g., duration of PTA, coma). The severity of the injury appears to hold the most weight with respect to prognosis for recovery. Several additional factors also require mentioning in this regard. These include age at the time of injury, rate of recovery, and premorbid functioning of the child and/or family,

Age at Time of Injury

As discussed earlier, it is clear that a traumatic brain injury may disrupt new learning along with a variety of other related neurocognitive functions. It has been speculated that younger children may be at greater risk for learning difficulties in that most of their learning is new. In general, these difficulties are related to the physiological maturity of the developing brain and to the functional status of the brain at the time of the injury. Consequently, age-dependent differences not only might be seen in the loss or change in functional status, but also in the recovery of functions (Fletcher et al., 1987).

For example, studies of children at least 5 years of age have noted that age at the time of injury was unrelated to either the severity of the neurocognitive sequelae or the rate of recovery (Chadwick et al., 1981; Klonoff et al., 1977; Levin & Eisenberg, 1979a). Studies including infants and preschoolers, however, have reported the presence of more severe long-term neurocognitive deficiencies in these children (Brink et al., 1970;

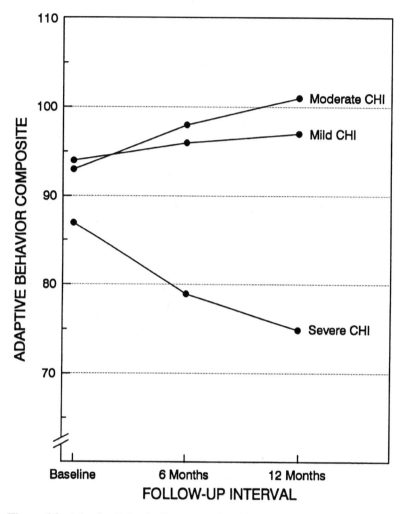

Figure 4.2. Adaptive Behavior Patterns at 6 and 12 Months Postinjury in Three Groups of Children With Closed Head Injury.
SOURCE: Fletcher, Ewing-Cobbs, Miner, Levin, and Eisenberg (1990). Reprinted with permission.

Ewing-Cobbs, Fletcher, Levin, Copeland, Francis, & Miner, 1994; Lange-Cosack, Wider, Schlesner, Grumme, & Kubicki, 1979; Shaffer et al., 1980).

Recovery Rates

As described earlier in this chapter, the rate and amount of recovery appear to be dependent, at least in part, upon the severity of the traumatic brain injury. In general, individuals incurring more severe injuries tend to evidence a slower rate of recovery than individuals who sustained mild or, in some instances, moderate traumatic brain injuries. Furthermore, it has been suggested that the more rapidly that any specific function emerges following an injury, the better the prognosis for that function (Roberts, 1979).

For adults and children, it seems that the major portion of recovery occurs during the first year following the injury (Brink et al., 1970; Klonoff et al., 1977), perhaps due to spontaneous remission or the specific interventions attempted. More specifically, Chadwick et al. (1981) demonstrated that most of the recovery that occurred tended to occur for more severely injured children. This conjecture is nicely illustrated in Figure 4.3 using their data from the Performance IQ on the Wechsler Intelligence Scale for Children. As can be seen, there was relatively little improvement in Performance IQ for their controls and mildly injured individuals at the 1-year and 30-month follow-up points. In contrast, however, there was significant improvement in Performance IQ by their severely injured group at the 1-year follow-up point, with some modest improvements continuing out to the 30-month point. Klonoff et al. (1977) even have shown that neuropsychological improvement can continue to be evidenced over a 5-year period.

Fletcher et al. (1987) and Taylor (1984) posited three different scenarios for age effects in a traumatic brain injury and subsequent recovery of function: (a) children show an increased vulnerability to damage, but less recovery of function than adults; (b) children evidence greater behavioral sparing and recovery of function than adults; and (c) the effects of a traumatic brain injury depend on the age of the child/adolescent, and recovery depends on the capacity of the developing brain to evolve alternate coping/behavioral strategies. Although the field has not yet arrived at clear answers with respect to these positions, it is clear that the increased precision in how traumatic brain injuries are classified will contribute to our understanding of how age at the time of injury affects ultimate outcome.

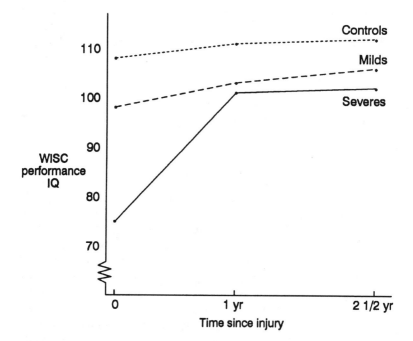

Figure 4.3. An Example of Recovery of Cognitive Functions Following Orthopedic and Head Injury in Children at 1 year- and 2½-Month Postinjury Intervals.
SOURCE: Chadwick, Rutter, Brown, Shaffer, and Traub (1981). Reprinted with permission.

Premorbid Functioning

Despite the epidemiological features discussed in Chapter 1 (e.g., more boys than girls sustaining traumatic brain injuries; more injuries occurring in lower socioeconomic status homes), and in contrast to the similar gender differences typically found in clinical samples of learning and psychiatric disorders, the gender of a child does not appear to affect the ultimate outcome (Chadwick, Rutter, Brown, 1981; Shaffer et al., 1980). Likewise, social class seems to exert little influence on outcome from a traumatic brain injury (Chadwick, Rutter, Brown, 1981), although clinical intuition persists in suggesting that children from more affluent backgrounds tend to show better improvement following an injury. Despite these findings, preinjury difficulties, particularly in the psychiatric domain, have proven to be predictive of later problems (Brown et al., 1981). These findings suggest the importance of gaining a clear and comprehensive preinjury history when working with children and adolescents who have sustained a traumatic brain injury.

SUMMARY

In this chapter, we provided an overview of the neurocognitive and psychosocial outcomes of pediatric traumatic brain injuries. As can be seen from this discussion, there is a multitude of neurocognitive and psycho-social deficits that can emerge following a traumatic brain injury. Further-more, there seems to be a trend for more significant and persistent neurocognitive sequelae in children and adolescents sustaining a severe traumatic brain injury, compared to children sustaining milder injuries.

The neurocognitive and psychosocial residuals for children with mild or even moderate brain injuries seems to be less clear, although when brain injuries of these severity levels do produce neurocognitive difficulties, recovery tends to occur over a briefer duration of time. Although children with severe injuries generally tend to have poorer prognoses, it is clear that individuals who have sustained milder types of head injury do show neurocognitive residuals, even if only for several months after the injury. Nonetheless, even these transient changes in neurobehavioral functioning can affect a child's social, academic, and family functioning, and the evolution of recent legislation (i.e., IDEA legislation) would appear to be beneficial to these children. Furthermore, given the timing of the injury (e.g., in regions of the country showing seasonal variations, most injuries tend to occur during the spring and summer months), it is likely that even a short recovery curve of 6 months could stretch over 2 school years and disrupt a child's academic progress quite significantly. Special education services would appear to be an efficient means for addressing the transient as well as more permanent deficits that can be seen with all types of trau-matic brain injury.

Additional issues related to the premorbid functioning status of the child and family and the age of the child also seem to impact upon ulti-mate outcomes. It remains unclear, however, how these factors interact to influence ultimate outcome from a traumatic brain injury. It should be recognized that research in pediatric traumatic brain injury is only in its beginning stages. Longitudinal studies comparing different types of injuries with respect to ultimate outcomes and employing more specific types of assessment are sorely needed in this field.

Part III

Assessment and Treatment

5

NEUROLOGICAL AND NEURODIAGNOSTIC TECHNIQUES

The majority of children and adolescents who suffer traumatic brain injury receive some degree of medical workup. The procedure selected generally depends on the medical severity of the case involved. These diagnostic workups allow the physician and other health professionals to decide the direction of treatment. They also may be useful with predicting long-term functional outcomes for injured children and adolescents. The purpose of this chapter is to give an overview of various neurological and neurodiagnostic techniques, the results of which frequently are included in case materials for a referred individual. The utility of these techniques in the diagnosis and treatment of TBI will be discussed.

NEUROLOGICAL EXAM
AND COMA RATING SCALE

Children and adolescents who have sustained a traumatic brain injury typically will initially be seen by a physician who may conduct a basic neurological evaluation. The extent of this exam will relate to the severity of the injury as well as to what other neurodiagnostic techniques may be utilized. For example, it may not be necessary to conduct an extensive neurological exam with a child or adolescent who has sustained a severe TBI, as other neurodiagnostic techniques are routinely ordered. On the other hand, a more comprehensive neurological exam may be conducted with the mild-to-moderate TBI to determine the extent to which further and more costly neurodiagnostic techniques may be needed.

Menkes (1990) emphasized several factors that should be assessed in a neurological examination of a child or adolescent with TBI. He suggested focusing on the state and quality of consciousness of the patient, possibly including traditional coma indices. Menkes (1990) also emphasized the importance of pupillary size and response to light. In addition, the examination should focus on symmetry of spontaneous movements and presence of various reflex responses. Measures of blood pressure, pulse, and respiration are also critical values to be obtained during the initial neurological evaluation. Menkes (1990) further advocated the importance of conducting these evaluations, particularly the level of consciousness and motor activity exams, at serial intervals, as serial examinations enable determining as to what further neurodiagnostic techniques and/or surgical interventions may be necessary.

Bruce and Zimmermann (1989) discussed the importance of the physical examination in the differential diagnosis of potential abuse with infants. These authors focused on the "shaken baby syndrome" and the difficulty there may be in a correct diagnosis of this condition. One factor these investigators emphasized is an examination of the optic fundi, important for the diagnosis of retinal hemorrhages, common injuries associated with violent shaking. They feel that the presence of retinal hemorrhages, in the absence of significant other trauma, is an important diagnostic observation for recognizing this syndrome.

Following initial neurological examination, most children or adolescents with TBI are rated on the Glasgow Coma Scale to determine severity of head injury. Although this is a commonly used technique, Lieh-Lai et al. (1992) questioned the predictive value of the Glasgow Coma Scale for children with traumatic brain injury. These authors utilized a sample of 79 children who had sustained varying degrees of TBI. Twenty-eight percent of the sample had initial Glasgow Coma Scale scores from 3 to 5, 36.7% had scores between 6 and 10, and 35.3% had scores between 11 and 13. The investigators followed many of these children with respect to their recovery process. In general, it was found that those children with low Glasgow Coma Scales (i.e., scores of 3 to 5) often did show favorable outcomes. It was noted that these children did require more aggressive therapy and did have a longer recovery period. They also found that hypoxic-ischemic insult was suggestive of a poorer outcome for children, regardless of level on the Glasgow Coma Scale. In general, the authors concluded that a significantly low Glasgow Coma Scale level is not always suggestive of a poor outcome; children with a severe head injury may require more intense therapy and aggressive treatment, but can still show significant recovery of function.

ELECTROENCEPHALOGRAPHY AND EVOKED POTENTIALS

Electrophysiological studies with traumatic-brain-injured children and adolescents often can provide important diagnostic or treatment information. The electroencephalograph (EEG) is a tool used to diagnose seizure disorders as well as other electrophysiological abnormalities. With adult populations, the EEG has demonstrated importance in monitoring severe head injuries. This technique has shown sensitivity to different hemispheric lesions as well as functional changes in brain activity (Schoenhuber & Gentilini, 1986). The EEG also has shown utility in the identification of subtle electrophysiological deficits following mild head injury (e.g., Courjon, 1972).

Clinical and research data suggest the diagnostic utility of the EEG with children and adolescents who have sustained a TBI. Mizrahi and Kellaway (1984) found a relationship between EEG abnormalities and severity of head injury. There have been little supportive data, however, with regard to early EEG signs being predictive of development of posttraumatic epilepsy (Jennett, 1975). In any event, routine EEGs often are requested for children and adolescents who have sustained a TBI. This is done to monitor electrophysiological activity, with a particular focus on detection of possible seizure activity.

Another form of electrophysiological diagnosis is through evoked potentials. These techniques measure the response of the central nervous system to selected external stimuli. There are a number of evoked potential paradigms; the visual evoked responses (VER), brain stem auditory evoked responses (BEAR), and somata-sensory evoked potentials (SEP) are the most commonly used in pediatric neurology (Menkes, 1990).

The VER paradigm involves flash stimuli presentation to the patient with the amplitude and latencies from the occipital lobe regions being recorded. The VER has proven to be useful in diagnosis of various types of central nervous system disorders with children. The technique also may be utilized with infants (Menkes, 1990). Little research, however, is available regarding the utility of the VER for children and adolescents with TBI.

The BEAR technique has gained clinical utility. This paradigm involves presentation of several clicks delivered to one ear that sequentially activate various cranial nerves and subsequently travel up through the brain stem. Amplitude and interpeak latencies are examined to determine the functional integrity of the brain stem auditory system. This technique can be utilized in diagnosis of hypoxic-anoxic disorders that may be secondary to traumatic brain injury, and it also can be prognostic with patients who are comatose secondary to severe TBI (Menkes, 1990).

The SEP method also provides information concerning interrelated areas of the central nervous system. This paradigm relies on stimulation of peripheral sensory nerves and examination of responses throughout the central nervous system. This technique involves the presentation of electrical stimulation to various parts of the skin and subsequent examination of interpeak latencies (Menkes, 1990). This method also may be useful in monitoring progress of comatose patients as well as with diagnosis of other disorders.

Little research is available concerning specific use of evoked potentials with children and adolescents with TBI. A recent study reported by Cusumano et al. (1992) examined evoked potential paradigms with comatose patients. Their sample did include several children and adolescents, as the age range was from 5 to 64 years. These authors found that use of various electrophysiological paradigms was predictive for their TBI patients. In particular, they found the SEP method to be the most reliable. These authors noted that examination of patterns emanating from the frontal areas was particularly predictive of central nervous system dysfunction.

EEG and evoked potentials provide information concerning electrophysiological activity within the central nervous system. Other diagnostic techniques indicate structural abnormalities, specific lesions within the brain, or secondary complications. The two most commonly used techniques for these types of information are computed tomography (CT) and magnetic resonance imaging (MRI).

COMPUTED TOMOGRAPHY

Computed tomography, originally introduced by Hounsfield (1973), is a means of detecting slight differences in density within the central nervous system. The technique involves radiation presented by a thin x-ray beam that is moved across the head (or other body part). Readings are obtained throughout the process and are fed into a computer that in turn calculates absorption coefficients for different areas of the brain. As indicated by Menkes (1990), most standard machines allow serial cuts of 10 mm thick, although the thickness can be reduced. The total radiation dose for a CT scan is somewhat less than that produced by a routine skull series. The entire procedure takes approximately 30 minutes and can be done with or without contrast substances. The contrast substances may be utilized to enhance resolution of various structures. The CT scan represents one of the most commonly used neurodiagnostic techniques for patients with traumatic brain injury (Mills et al., 1986).

A primary use of CT scans for patients with traumatic brain injury is for identification of hematomas and other secondary complications that may require immediate medical intervention. Esparza et al. (1985) discussed the utility of repeated CT scans for medical management of children who had sustained a severe TBI. The sample for their study included 56 children with Glasgow Coma Scale scores of less than 8 upon admission to the emergency room. A CT scan was performed upon admission, 3 days later, and then at variable intervals. These authors felt the CT scan studies were effective at showing the presence of extradural and subdural hematomas. They also were able to diagnose various cortical contusions and possible diffuse axonal shearing. With regard to outcome, these investigators found children with extradural hematomas showed the most benign profile with regard to residual deficits. Presence of diffuse axonal shearing was predictive of a less favorable outcome. These investigators argued for the importance of utilizing serial CT examinations during the acute phase.

Sganzerla et al. (1989) utilized CT scans to manage treatment for children with severe traumatic brain injury. This study utilized a sample of 41 children who had sustained a significant traumatic brain injury. The investigators used CT scans to identify the presence of either diffuse axonal injury (DAI) or diffuse brain swelling (DBS). DAI was diagnosed when there were midline hemorrhages or multiple small hemorrhages seen on the CT scans, or when no detectable brain abnormalities were noted on the serial CTs, but there was immediate loss of consciousness followed by a prolonged coma. DBS was diagnosed via CT showing narrowing or obliteration of the ventricles and/or basal cisterns. The results of the scan showed a relatively even distribution of DAI and DBS. Twenty of the children (48.8%) showed indications of DAI; 51.2% of the sample had evidence of DBS. The CT scans also showed evidence of intracranial pressure, which was monitored and treated in 8 of the children. In general, the authors found that intracranial hypertension was associated with a more negative outcome for the children in their sample.

In summary, CT scans do appear to be effective in identification of certain types of hematomas (e.g., Esparza et al., 1985; Kang, Park, Kim, Kim, & Song, 1989). The technique appears to be particularly useful when used in a serial fashion (Cooper, Maravilla, & Moody, 1979; Esparza et al., 1985; Sganzerla et al., 1989). Although the CT scan is a critical diagnostic tool in the management of pediatric TBI, there may be instances when other types of information are needed. In this regard, the physician may order a magnetic resonance imaging study.

MAGNETIC RESONANCE IMAGING

Magnetic resonance imaging (MRI) is another noninvasive neurodiagnostic procedure. The physical principles of MRI are beyond the scope of this text (interested readers should consult texts such as Brant-Zawadzki & Norman, 1987). The advent of MRI has provided yet another valuable neurodiagnostic tool for both pediatric and adult patients. MRI is superior to CT at diagnosis of various types of tumors as well as providing specific information concerning demyelinization. The technique also has proven useful in the identification of specific cortical changes including micropolygyri, lissencephaly, or heterotopic gray matter (Menkes, 1990).

MRI is an extremely useful tool for gathering information on children and adolescents with TBI. Levin et al. (1989) utilized MRI for more precise identification and diagnosis of shaken baby syndrome, and noted that MRI studies can detect small cerebral hemorrhages in the infant (e.g., Gomori, Grossman, & Goldberg, 1985). Levin et al. (1989) reported findings for a specific case study where there was the suspicion of shaken baby syndrome. The CT scan for this infant was within normal limits. MRI, however, revealed several hemorrhages and a subdural hematoma. These authors concluded that MRI studies are extremely useful in identifying small lesions that may not be detected by CT scans or other procedures.

Sato et al. (1989) examined the use of MRI for children with TBI. This study described 19 cases of children being investigated for trauma believed to be secondary to physical abuse. All of the children underwent both CT scans and MRI studies. Thirteen of the patients presented with identified intracranial abnormalities on both the CT and MRI images; three patients showed no abnormalities with either procedure. Three other patients demonstrated abnormalities only on the MRI studies. These investigators found the CT scan to be superior to the MRI for identification of subarachnoid hemorrhages, whereas the MRI studies seemed to be more effective at imaging subdural hematomas, bland contusions, and shearing injuries. The MRI was also superior in demonstrating nonhemorrhagic foci throughout the brain structure. Sato et al. (1989) reported findings that showed the MRI to be more sensitive to detecting potential ages of hematomas. These investigators felt that this was particularly important in that it may provide clues to children who may be subjected to abuse over an extended period of time, and more generally, to distinguish older brain injuries from newer ones.

The advent of MRI has significantly increased the diagnostic capacities available to physicians. MRI seems to be particularly effective at demonstrating and localizing extra-axial and intra-axial traumatic lesions (Alexander, Schor, & Smith, 1986; Gentry, Godersky, Thompson, & Dunn, 1988). The technique also appears to be superior to CT in showing nonhemorrhagic foci as well as potential shearing of connective white tissue. Recent computer technology has allowed construction of three-dimensional images of the brain based on MRI. These factors all contribute to more effective medical management of children and adolescents with TBI, as well as providing important neuroanatomical information that may be predictive of functional outcomes.

SUMMARY

Recent advances in neurodiagnostics and neuroimaging have contributed to the remarkable progress with treatment of TBI children and adolescents. Physicians have a variety of techniques at their disposal to not only establish the severity of the injury, but also help monitor changes that can dictate the need for various medical procedures. This chapter has outlined different neurodiagnostic procedures, from basic neurological exams to more complex MRI studies. With these procedures, along with such scales as the Glasgow Coma Scale, it is possible to rate the initial severity of a TBI. CT scans are useful, particularly because of their demonstrated sensitivity to many types of hematomas. MRI studies can further facilitate diagnosis as this procedure shows more subtle hematomas as well as provides specific information concerning diffuse injuries, particularly with connective white tissue. These various techniques are one aspect of the treatment and care of the child or adolescent with TBI. Another important factor is the cognitive and behavioral sequelae secondary to the injury. This is described through a comprehensive neuropsychological evaluation, which is the focus of the next chapter.

6

NEUROPSYCHOLOGICAL ASSESSMENT

To facilitate the transition of the child or adolescent with TBI to different environments, it is necessary to evaluate cognitive functions. A comprehensive evaluation allows the pediatric neuropsychologist to formulate a profile of cognitive strengths and weaknesses, and to initiate appropriate intervention strategies. This chapter will focus on the neuropsychological evaluation process. It is important to note that it is critical that the neuropsychologist work with other professionals. An effective transition for most children and adolescents with TBI is accomplished best through an interdisciplinary team approach. Assessment data collected by the pediatric neuropsychologist allow for effective communication with other professionals as well as with parents and primary caregivers. This chapter will outline the assessment process, with particular emphasis on assessment of neuropsychological constructs. Although these constructs should not be viewed as orthogonal, as clear interrelationships exist (e.g., attention and memory), they will be discussed independently as a teaching heuristic. Issues relevant to interpretation also are presented.

ASSESSMENT PROCESS

Collection of Background Information

The initial phase of a comprehensive neuropsychological evaluation should be collection and review of important background information. Records relevant to the injury and subsequent hospitalization should be examined. This review should focus on factors discussed in earlier chapters, specifically, neurodiagnostic measures, length of coma, and approximate length of posttraumatic amnesia. Hospital notes (if available) should be reviewed for information concerning level of agitation or confusion as well as rehabilitative services that may have been initiated in the acute setting.

It is particularly important for information to be gathered concerning specific medications on which the child or adolescent has been placed. As indicated by Aicardi (1987), children and adolescents who have sustained some type of brain injury are at higher risk for epilepsy. As a result, children and adolescents with traumatic brain injury are frequently placed on some type of anticonvulsant medication. The pediatric neuropsychologist and other professionals needs to be aware of these medications as some of these can influence performance on particular cognitive testing.

Corbett and Trimble (1983) reviewed the possible adverse side effects of anticonvulsants. Several studies reviewed by these investigators indicated cerebellar-type dysfunction associated with toxic levels of phenytoin. They also noted potential negative side effects associated with carbamazepine. Some studies suggest the negative cognitive side effects are associated with anticonvulsant medication, but many other studies indicate positive effects with medicines that are well regulated. In general, the literature suggests high or toxic blood levels to be the most important factor that can negatively impact cognitive functions (Rodin, Schmaltz, Maltz, & Twitty, 1986). There also are indications that polydrug therapy can have negative effects, either directly or synergistically, on cognitive development and selected cognitive processes (Bennett-Levy & Stores, 1984).

The factors associated with side effects and use of anticonvulsants, as well as other medications, suggest that the pediatric neuropsychologist should maintain close contact with the prescribing physician. A dialogue needs to be maintained between these professionals to provide detailed patient observations, patient subjective reports, and an accurate estimate of current functioning. The prescribing physician should indicate to the evaluator when the child or adolescent is stable on his or her current medication regime. The pediatric neuropsychologist may not have the luxury to delay testing, but should incorporate medical information to draw more meaningful conclusions.

In addition to reviewing current medical records, it is imperative that the pediatric neuropsychologist review premorbid medical history. This should focus on information concerning any preexisting neurological history that could influence current testing results, such as a previous head injury, history of seizures, or history of other neurological complications. It also is important to obtain information concerning other medical conditions that can have a direct or indirect impact on cognitive processes. History of premorbid psychiatric difficulties also should be obtained (this will be discussed further in Chapter 7).

Along with reviews of current and past medical status, the pediatric neuropsychologist should obtain other important background information. This should include a comprehensive developmental history, encompassing the mother's report of pregnancy and delivery, and use of tobacco, alcohol, or other drugs during pregnancy. A review of the family history also is important in that it allows mapping of familial trends such as learning difficulties or associated attention problems. Other critical information to obtain during the preassessment phase are developmental milestones and school history. Whenever possible, data concerning motor and language development should be obtained to determine the presence of delays or deficits prior to the accident. Comprehensive school records should be obtained and reviewed, including previous testing, school attendance, and factors such as grade retention or placement in special education classes.

In many cases, much of this information may not be available immediately or at all. In such cases, demographic information has been suggested as useful in gaining an estimate of preinjury level of cognitive functioning (i.e., IQ). For example, Barona, Reynolds, and Chastain (1984) provided such a model to predict premorbid WAIS-R IQs by using the variables of age, race, gender, education, occupation, and type of residence. The values for each of these demographic variables and the resultant equations can be seen in Table 6.1.

Similarly, Reynolds and Gutkin (1979) developed a set of equations to predict WISC-R IQs, which can be seen in Table 6.2. The use of demographic data to predict premorbid cognitive functioning holds much promise, particularly as they can be used regardless of a patient's condition; however, it is important to combine these demographic equations with other tangible information (e.g., grades) to describe premorbid functioning more fully (Crawford, in press). Furthermore, these procedures tend to underestimate the premorbid functioning of brighter individuals (i.e., Full Scale IQ > 120), and overestimate the functioning of lower functioning individuals (i.e., Full Scale IQ < 69). A set of equations for the WISC-III or WPPSI-R has not yet been developed.

TABLE 6.1 Regression Equations and Standard Error of Estimates for WAIS-R IQs

Estimated Verbal IQ = 54.23 + 0.49 (age) + 1.92 (sex) + 4.24 (race) + 5.25 (education) + 1.89 (occupation) + 1.24 (urban-rural residence). Standard error of estimate of VIQ = 11.79; R = .62.

Estimated Performance IQ = 61.58 + 0.31 (age) + 1.09 (sex) + 4.95 (race) + 3.75 (education) + 1.54 (occupation) + .82 (region). Standard error of estimate of PIQ = 13.23; R = .49.

Estimated Full Scale IQ = 54.96 + 0.47 (age) + 1.76 (sex) + 4.71 (race) + 5.05 (education) + 1.89 (occupation) + .59 (region). Standard error of estimate of FSIQ = 12.14; R = .60.

For each equation, demographic variables take the following values:

Sex: Female = 1; Male = 2

Race: White = 3; Black = 2; Other = 1

Occupation: Professional/Technical = 6; Managerial/Official/Clerical/Sales = 5; Skilled Labor = 4; Not in Labor Force = 3; Semiskilled labor = 2; Unskilled labor = 1

Region: Southern = 1; North Central = 2; Western = 3; Northeast = 4

Residence: Rural = 1; Urban = 2

Age: 16-17 = 1; 18-19 = 2; 20-24 = 3; 25-34 = 4; 35-44 = 5; 45-54 = 6; 55-64 = 7; 65-69 = 8; 70-74 = 9

Education: 0-7 = 1; 8 = 2; 9-11 = 3; 12 = 4; 13-15 = 5; 16+=6

SOURCE: Adapted from Barona, Reynolds, and Chastain (1984).

The purpose of this initial phase is to obtain and integrate all available background information. This allows the pediatric neuropsychologist to formulate an estimate concerning premorbid functioning for the child or adolescent. It also allows the professional to determine possible associated factors that can influence the assessment procedure itself. After collecting data, the pediatric neuropsychologist is ready to begin the comprehensive individual assessment procedure.

Assessment of Intellectual and Academic Skills

A major component of the overall battery conducted by the pediatric neuropsychologist is the traditional psychoeducational evaluation. This, at a minimum, involves the administration of a general intellectual measure and assessment of academic abilities. This component is important for consultation with schools, and it also plays a key role in the diagnostic aspects of the neuropsychological battery. The patterns yielded on measures of intellectual ability as well as academic skills can provide useful information concerning cognitive strengths and weaknesses. These obser-

TABLE 6.2 Regression Equations and Standard Error of Estimates for WISC-R IQs

Estimated Verbal IQ = 127.85 − 3.7 (SES) − 8.86 (race) − 2.40 (sex) − 0.68 (region) − 1.16 (residence).

Standard error of estimate for VIQ = 13.47.

Estimated Performance IQ = 121.08 − 9.18 (race) − 2.80 (SES) − 1.07 (residence) − 0.64 (sex).

Standard error of estimate for PIQ = 13.97.

Estimated Full Scale IQ = 126.9 − 3.65 (SES) − 9.72 (race) − 1.79 (sex) − 1.20 (residence) − 0.41 (region).

Standard error of estimate for FSIQ = 13.50.

For each equation, demographic variables take the following values:

Sex: Male = 1; Female = 2

Race: White = 1; Black = 2; Other = 3

SES (see Wechsler, 1974, for classification details): Upper Class = 1; Upper-middle = 2; Middle = 3; Lower-middle = 4; Lower = 5

Region (see Wechsler, 1974, for classification details): Northeast = 1; Northcentral = 2; South = 3; West = 4

Residence: Urban = 1; Rural = 2

SOURCE: Adapted from Reynolds and Gutkin (1979).

vations then can be utilized to formulate diagnostic decisions as well as more effective intervention strategies.

As mentioned in Chapter 4, verbal intellectual abilities tend to recover at a more rapid rate than performance abilities (e.g., Chadwick, Rutter, Shaffer et al., 1981; Levin & Benton, 1986). Serial assessments do, however, indicate recovery of performance abilities (Chadwick, Rutter, Brown et al., 1981). This recovery pattern needs to be considered in interpreting results from intellectual assessments. Although the traditional view would suggest depressed performance relative to verbal skills to be attributable to more nonverbal/visuospatial deficits, other factors may play a role with regard to children and adolescents who have sustained a traumatic brain injury.

Bawden et al. (1985) examined speed of performance in children who had sustained a closed head injury. As these investigators point out, previous literature had indicated that head-injured patients showed slowed reaction times and deficits in speeded performance (Klonoff, 1971; Winogron et al., 1984). In this investigation, Bawden et al. (1985) examined skills across head injury severity levels. They divided their subjects into mildly, moderately, and severely injured groups. They conducted comprehensive retrospective examinations to exclude children with severe behavioral or neurological problems prior to their head injury. As part of the overall battery, the children were administered selected subtests from the WISC-R. This included Coding, Block Design, Object Assembly, Picture Completion, and Picture Arrangement. The Coding subtest was classified as highly speeded whereas the other WISC-R subtests were in the moderately speeded category. The overall results indicated the severely injured group to be significantly lower on Performance Scale IQ. In examining the pattern for the individual subtests, significant differences were found on Coding, Picture Completion, and Block Design. The severely injured group was significantly more impaired on these measures compared with the other two groups. No significant differences were found on Picture Arrangement or Object Assembly. Those in the severe head injury group did not show generalized deficits in basic motor function or visuospatial abilities, but they did show deficits on tasks requiring motor speed, as well as motor speed and visual/spatial integration skills.

The results of this study suggest the need to account for speeded mental processing when interpreting results of intellectual measures. This appears to be particularly important with children who have sustained a severe head injury. Although the Wechsler scales are generally the measure of choice, this slowed mental processing needs to be accounted for when interpreting Performance Scale IQ scores. If the pediatric neuropsychologist is interested in assessing nonverbal reasoning abilities when time is not a factor, limit testing on the WISC-III can be conducted (e.g., deleting time limits on various subtests) or other intellectual measures should be considered (e.g., Kaufman Brief Intelligence Test, Kaufman & Kaufman, 1990; Matrix Analogies Test, Naglieri, 1985; Wechsler Adult Intelligence Scale—Revised NI; Kaplan, Fein, Morris, & Delis, 1991).

The function of the general intellectual measure should not only be to provide a profile of cognitive strengths and weaknesses, but also to yield an overall intellectual level that can then serve as a possible bench mark for comparison of other results. From a psychometric viewpoint, the Full Scale IQ score yielded by intellectual measures is the most reliable and valid. Examination of subtest scatter as well as patterns within individual scales is extremely useful from a clinical and neuropsychological standpoint, but can be somewhat risky from a psychometric standpoint. This is

particularly the case when subtests do not contain enough subtest speci-
ficity. Consequently, the role of the general intellectual measure should
be first and foremost an indicator of overall intellectual abilities. Furthermore, the comparison between verbal and nonverbal domains (e.g.,
Wechsler Scales) can prove useful in mapping recovery of function. Long-
term follow-up using these scales also can provide important information
concerning residual deficits.

The next phase of the neuropsychological evaluation should involve
administration of academic measures. Because most children and adolescents are transitioned back into the school environment, it is important for
information concerning academic strengths and weaknesses to be provided to school officials. As mentioned above, patterns of academic skills
also can provide useful diagnostic information.

In selecting an assessment of academic skills, it is critical for the measure
to be comprehensive. A screening of academic abilities (e.g., WRAT-3)
can provide informative guidelines, but more comprehensive assessment tools often are indicated. Ewing-Cobbs et al. (1987) found that written-
language abilities appear to be particularly susceptible following traumatic
brain injury in children. These investigators felt that written language is
particularly vulnerable in children because this is an emerging skill that
is not well consolidated. The types of errors noted with their sample of
head-injured children included omissions, misspellings, and capitaliza-
tion errors. They felt that these errors reflected a more generalized deficit
secondary to attention and organizational deficiencies rather than difficulties with fundamental semantic, syntactic, or apraxic deficits.

No matter what measure is selected, it is imperative for the pediatric
neuropsychologist to conduct a comprehensive error analysis. Even the
most basic academic scales can be examined for error types. This should
include review of misspellings to determine phonetic accuracy, breakdowns
in math calculation abilities, as well as the child's ability to phonetically
decode words not readily available in their sight word vocabulary. Examining the specific error types as well as the global scores allows for a more
comprehensive intervention plan and it may yield important diagnostic
findings.

Lastly, as noted in Chapter 4, it is crucial to make the distinction between a child's performance on an individually administered achievement test
and in the classroom. For example, in an older child or adolescent, basic
academic skills may appear intact. It would be a mistake, however, to

assume that these intact skill levels translate into a commensurate performance level in the classroom. Individual achievement testing typically provides the structure and time for a child to perform well, and these tests do tend to tap old, perhaps previously automatized, knowledge. The rapid retrieval, organization, attention, and other functions required to perform adequately in the classroom setting may be the very deficits that many children with TBI have incurred, and these contribute to lowering performance levels in the classroom or other settings. Care should be taken to evaluate a child or adolescent for these differing levels of performance. A call to a teacher, a behavior rating scale, or a portfolio assessment can be helpful in this regard.

Assessment of Motor and Sensory Functions

Assessment of motor functions is an integral part of traditional neuropsychological testing. Most batteries incorporate some measure of psychomotor speed, motor strength, and motor coordination. These types of assessments are useful in determining level and pattern (i.e., lateralization) of dysfunction.

Specific motor deficits have been described for children and adolescents with traumatic brain injury. In more severe cases, a hemiparesis or quadraparesis may be evident. Often, however, children and adolescents show motor difficulties that tend to resolve, usually within 6 months following the injury (Fuld & Fisher, 1977). Other types of deficits that have been noted, particularly with younger children, include problems with fine motor coordination, difficulties with motor integration, tremors, and problems with rapid alternating movements (Dimitrijevic, Dimitrijevic, Kinalski, McKay, & Sherwood, 1987; Rourke, Fisk, & Strang, 1986).

In evaluating motor functions, it is important not only to look for noticeable dysfunction, such as tremors or hemiparesis, but also to examine asymmetry of performance. Children and adolescents should evidence a dominant-hand advantage of about 10% to 20% on all motor tasks (Spreen & Gaddes, 1969). Dominant-hand advantages of less than 10% or a nondominant-hand advantage are often suggestive of lateralized dysfunction in the dominant hemisphere. In addition, an advantage of greater than 20% may be indicative of residual deficits greater in the nondominant hemisphere. For children and adolescents who have sustained significant brain injury, motor speed differences may be present initially, but often resolve with time. Care should be taken to rule out the presence of peripheral nerve injuries, as these can impact motor strength, speed, and coordination. Similarly, cerebellar injuries have same-side as opposed to contralateral implications.

In assessing motor functions, it is important that the pediatric neuro-psychologist observe for qualitative signs of dysfunction, including asso-ciated movements or movements of extremities not involved with the motor task. Persistence of such extracurricular movements beyond age 10 often suggests dysfunction with the motor inhibitory system.

Examination of sensory functions also can yield important diagnostic in-formation. As with motor functions, perhaps the most telling diagnostic factor with tactile perception is lateral comparisons. Significant differ-ences between the right and the left side can indicate where more residual deficits are lateralized, particularly in the posterior parietal cortical re-gion. Tactile kinesthetic functions are easy to examine with tasks that do not require a great deal of time. Tests such as graphasthesia (recognition of shapes, letters, or numbers drawn on the hands) and stereognosis (recog-nition of objects by touch) can yield information concerning tactile discrimi-nation and tactile integration functions. Yet another means to examine tactile functions is with finger localization and fingertip symbol or number writing.

As with motor functions, dysfunction with tactile integration typically indicates damage to the contralateral hemisphere. Cautionary notes in exam-ining such functions are warranted. Although many tasks, such as fingertip number writing and stereognosis, do tap tactile kinesthetic functions, they also load on other factors. Other major factors that may influence perfor-mance on these tasks are focused and sustained attention. It is critical to conduct a thorough examination to determine if errors are strictly due to tactile integration, a combination of factors, or skills unrelated to tactile kinesthetic abilities. This may require the use of both formal and informal measures, and requires close observation on the part of the examiner.

Another sensory function that is critical to examine is visual-perceptual ability. Skills and abilities examined within this realm include visual per-ception, visual discrimination, and visual-spatial orientation abilities. Al-though there are a number of formal measures for each of these abilities, generalized assessments can yield important information in this realm. For example, many of the subtests from the Wechsler Performance Scale have visual-perceptual and visual-spatial components. Other tests are sensitive to visual sequencing abilities as well as visual-motor integration skills.

Examination of both tactile and visual perceptual abilities is important with regard to recommendations to school personnel. Clearly, visual-perceptual abilities are important for such skills as reading and writing, and are particularly critical for academic and social success of younger children. The academic relevance of tactile integration functions is less evident, but these functions do play a role in fine-motor control in handwriting and sensory-motor learning, and may serve as neurodevelopmental predictors of later academic problems. Furthermore, it may be important to communicate deficits in tactile perceptual abilities to a teacher if he or she is considering using a multimodel sensory approach.

Assessment of Speech/Language Functions

The susceptibility of speech/language dysfunction secondary to traumatic brain injury has been the focus of considerable interest. Some researchers contend there is a very high probability of language sequelae, whereas others have found no clear relationship between severity of head injury and persistent language dysfunction (Hecaen, 1976; Rothenberger, 1986). These data have been reviewed in Chapter 4. Despite the discrepancy in the available research literature, it is critical that speech and language functions be evaluated in children and adolescents who have sustained a traumatic brain injury. During the initial assessment, these abilities may be significantly affected secondary to such conditions as posttraumatic amnesia or disorientation and confusion. As these conditions begin to clear, the pediatric neuropsychologist should be able to gain a more accurate view concerning specific language processes.

Ewing-Cobbs et al. (1987) examined language abilities in children and adolescents who had sustained a traumatic brain injury. Their review of the literature suggested that oral fluency and naming abilities appear to be the most susceptible to pediatric traumatic brain injury. In their investigation of language functions, these investigators examined children and adolescents approximately 6 months after sustaining a traumatic brain injury. They examined two clinical groupings: mild and moderate/severe. Those subjects tested were administered a comprehensive battery of language functions. The overall results indicated that a very high percentage of this clinical sample did evidence significant language difficulties. Expressive abilities appeared to be more susceptible than did receptive functions. Functions most likely to be impaired were description of object function, repeating sentences, word fluency, writing to dictation, and copying sentences. Very little impairment was noted on measures of confrontational naming, sentence construction, and auditory comprehension of single words. When examined within categorical classifications, the moderate/ severe group did show a greater pattern of dysfunction, particularly on measures of expressive ability. The investigators noted that the language difficulties shown in these clinical samples were not specific in nature, nor did they vary consistently with laterality of cerebral involvement.

This investigation, as well as others, points toward the importance of incorporating assessment of language functions in an overall neuropsychological evaluation. It appears particularly critical to utilize measures of written language as well as oral-expressive ability. Receptive abilities do not appear to be particularly vulnerable, but it is still important to evaluate processes from this domain as they may provide vehicles for remediation. Although the pediatric neuropsychologist may have some knowledge with regard to general evaluations of expressive and receptive language abilities, it is recommended that a comprehensive evaluation from a speech/ language pathologist be obtained. These professionals have more expertise in evaluating the finer aspects of language functions as well as assessing pragmatic language abilities. The results of a comprehensive speech/ language evaluation also can facilitate interpretation of the neuropsychological assessment, particularly with aphasic/dysphasic patients.

Assessment of Memory Functions

Most syndromes involving brain dysfunction for children and adolescents as well as adults generally involve some impairment of memory functions. The literature on adults is fairly clear in indicating lateralization of memory functions, whereby left temporal dysfunction is more associated with verbal memory deficits, and right temporal lobe damage is associated more with nonverbal and visual memory dysfunction. This strong lateralization pattern is less specific for children, although there is some evidence to suggest less efficiency with learning of verbal material being associated with left hemisphere damage and impaired learning for nonverbal and visual material being associated with right hemisphere damage (Fedio & Mirsky, 1969).

Children and adolescents who have sustained a traumatic brain injury frequently demonstrate deficits in memory function. For example, utilizing the Selective Reminding Test, which is a measure of verbal memory and verbal learning Eisenberg, Levin, and Papanicolaou (1985) found persistent memory deficits in children; however, adolescents showed a stronger recovery rate.

In addition to generalized verbal memory deficits, researchers also have demonstrated deficits with recognition memory (Levin, Eisenberg, Wigg, & Kobayashi, 1982). Recognition memory deficits are usually associated with more severe head injury. In addition, Levin, Eisenberg et al. (1982) found less impairment with adolescents. They felt that adolescents may be less susceptible to recognition memory impairment because they are able to utilize more effective strategies.

In general, the literature suggests a variety of deficits with memory functions associated with traumatic brain injury. It appears particularly important to assess memory functions in children sustaining traumatic brain injuries as long-lasting deficits appear to be more persistent with this group, compared with adolescents. This is particularly the case with children who have suffered a severe head injury. The pediatric neuropsychologist may wish to select a battery and/or standardized measure of memory functions, but certain elements need to be included no matter how mnestic abilities are assessed. This includes measuring short-term recall, efficiency of encoding/consolidation of both verbal and visual material, delayed recall, and prospective memory functions. Recognition memory also should be screened in children and adolescents who have sustained mild-to-moderate head injuries. A more thorough assessment of recognition skills appears important with children who have sustained severe traumatic brain injury.

Assessment of Attention

As noted in Chapter 4, attentional problems for children and adolescents with TBI are very common. These deficits range from hyperactivity to poor concentration and decreased speed of performance. Given the research evidence, it is important to incorporate measures of attention in a neuropsychological assessment.

Attention is a complex network with various neurological substrates (Halperin, McKay, Matier, & Sharma, 1994). The pediatric neuropsychologist needs to focus on different levels of attention throughout the evaluation. This includes examination of arousal, vigilance/attention span, perseverance, distractibility, and inhibitory processes. These skills are best assessed through direct measures as well as qualitative observations. Documentation of attention deficits can be helpful in delineating various brain structures that may have residual damage as well as to provide information useful in formulating intervention strategies.

Assessment of Executive Functions

Evaluation of executive functions has not always received appropriate attention in pediatric populations. This may be attributed to developmental models that argued that the frontal lobes and prefrontal cortex do not fully mature until adolescence or early adulthood (Dennis, 1991). Current research findings, however, show that much of the frontal areas do mature during childhood.

As has been reported in Chapter 2, the frontal lobes are particularly susceptible to the effects of traumatic brain injury. Mateer and Williams (1991) presented four case studies of children who had sustained frontal lobe damage via a traumatic brain injury. Consistent findings reported across the subjects included initial problems with alertness, change in appetite/sleep, irritability, distractibility, impulsivity, social problems, attention difficulties, and academic production deficits. The investigators acknowledged that these children did sustain traumatic brain injury that likely produced damage to the frontal lobes and other areas as well, but they noted that the persistent deficits are well defined and consistent with a frontal lobe syndrome.

Dennis (1991) has presented a comprehensive model for the function and assessment of frontal lobe abilities with children and adolescents. This framework is hierarchical in nature, whereby initial stages comprise basic attention and orientation skills and subsequent stages include working memory/representational level, a metarepresentational level, and a monitoring system. The initial input operator stage is concerned with the regulation of intention. Other operations involved with this skill include vigilance, anticipatory set, and interference control. The next level (working memory) allows the child or adolescent to temporarily hold and manipulate information. This is a more complex skill that involves the processing of incoming information as well as the integration of already processed information. The next higher level involves what Dennis (1991) terms mental models. This term includes such factors as mental flexibility, shifting of attention and decision making, planning, sequencing, and inferential processing. Also within this realm are the monitoring systems that allow comparisons for incoming information with previously learned mental sets. Yet another level within Dennis's (1991) framework is semantic representation, which involves determining the meaning of words as well as discourse. At a higher level is metarepresentation, which enables the child or adolescent to make predictions based on the use and manipulation of obtained concepts. Dennis (1991) provides the specific means for as- sessing each of these levels and discusses the important role of frontal lobe functions with regard to cognitive abilities and social skills. She also em- phasizes the important developmental aspects of frontal lobe functions and the need to consider neurodevelopment when assessing these abilities.

As mentioned previously, the frontal lobes do appear to be particularly susceptible to injury in children and adolescents who have sustained traumatic brain injury. Snow (in press) investigated sequencing and mental flexibility in a sample of children with TBI. These children were compared with other clinical subsamples, which included children with spina bifida, children with specific learning disabilities, and children diagnosed with attention deficit hyperactivity disorder. The results indicated considerable variability for all groups, although the children with spina bifida were the most impaired. The children with TBI did show some difficulties with speeded mental processing and mental flexibility. These results are consistent with those discussed by Mateer and Williams (1991), suggesting possible frontal lobe involvement with this clinical sample.

Developmental studies as well as applied clinical research continue to advance our knowledge concerning executive processes in children and adolescents. As a result, it becomes more important and meaningful to administer measures of these functions to children and adolescents who have sustained traumatic brain injury. Although the pediatric neuropsychologist may not want to interpret these as strictly assessing "frontal lobe functions," it is imperative to include measures of attention, problem solving, mental flexibility, and planning in a comprehensive neuropsychological evaluation. Assessment of these functions becomes particularly important with older children and adolescents. In addition to psychoeducational and neuropsychological measures, evaluation of overt behavior as well as social interaction abilities are imperative to interpreting results. These issues will be discussed in the next chapter.

INTEGRATION
OF TEST RESULTS

The pediatric neuropsychologist needs to focus on a number of considerations when interpreting a neuropsychological profile for a child or adolescent with TBI. Figure 6.1 provides a schematic representation of the major phases of an evaluation. Furthermore, as noted in Figure 6.1, in addition to focusing on pattern of test scores, qualitative observations during the assessment procedure are critical. Observing and analyzing how the child problem-solves or makes errors provide diagnostic information, as well as data useful for generating more meaningful and ecologically valid intervention strategies. The qualitative findings allow the neuropsychologist to gain an increased understanding of the underlying etiology of test score patterns. For example, it may be that a child shows a rather generalized pattern of deficit, but the majority of the errors may be due to poor prob- lem solving or difficulties with sustained attention. This is not to discount the importance of quantitative test scores, as these are the psychometric indicators that best document recovery of function, but to encourage the use of both qualitative and quantitative findings in an evaluation.

Fletcher and Taylor (1984) presented a critical essay focusing on neuropsychological assessment in children. Although this important article is appropriate to all child and adolescent clinical populations, it is particularly germane for assessment of the patient with TBI. Fletcher and Taylor (1984) pointed out a number of fallacies that can impede meaningful interpretation of neuropsychological results in children. These fallacies include the assumption that procedures that are valuable with adults are just as sensitive to brain-related dysfunction with children; the assumption that tests designed and developed for adults measure the same skills for children; the belief that a behavioral deficit or learning problem, as opposed to a specific measure, is assumed to automatically signal difficulties with brain function; and overrepresentation of behavioral tests and/or observations. Fletcher and Taylor (1984) subsequently provided a more appropriate framework for pediatric neuropsychological assessment. The overriding emphasis of this model is to focus on developmental changes:

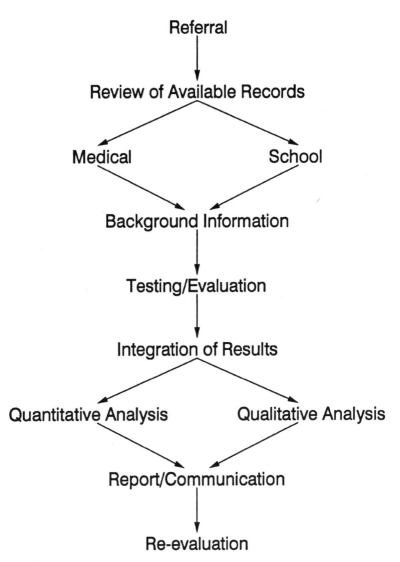

Figure 6.1. Primary Components of a Comprehensive Neuropsychological Evaluation.

TABLE 6.3 Evaluation Schedule for Traumatically Brain-Injured Children and Adolescents

Age/Severity	Schedule
7 or younger	Initial eval within 6 months
Mild/Moderate	Follow-up evals at 1-year intervals if necessary
7 or younger	Initial eval within 6 months
Severe	Follow-up evals at 6-month intervals for 3 years, extended to 1- to 3-year intervals
8 or older	Initial eval within 6 months
Mild/Moderate	Follow-up evals at 1- to 3-year intervals if necessary
8 or older	Initial eval within 6 months
Severe	Follow-up evals at 1-year intervals for 3 years, extended to 3-year intervals

"With change becoming the focal point for developmental neuropsychology, the questions addressed by researchers will likely shift. Questions about how childhood disabilities disrupt processes of change may begin to take precedence over the current pre-occupation with deficit brain areas" (p. 51). Focusing on developmental change is particularly important for the child or adolescent who has sustained a TBI.

Table 6.3 presents a proposed assessment schedule for children and adolescents who have sustained a traumatic brain injury. This model focuses on a number of key components, including severity of injury, age of onset, and a need for serial assessment. It is appropriate, particularly with younger children, that a serial assessment model be implemented. This allows the pediatric neuropsychologist to map recovery of function more accurately and to focus on interweaving developmental changes. This information allows determination of the extent to which acquired brain injury disrupts developmental processes and interferes with quantitative and qualitative changes in behavior. The assessment schedules presented in Table 6.3 are merely suggestions, and certainly there is room for flexibility. For example, it may not be necessary to assess younger children with severe traumatic brain injury with the frequency suggested by this model. On the other hand, there may be instances where children and adolescents who have sustained a mild-to-moderate head injury may show more severe deficits and therefore warrant more frequent reevaluations. It also should be noted that the assessment schedule does not call for a complete neuro-psychological evaluation at each testing period. The pediatric neuropsy-chologist may merely want to perform selected follow-up testing to ascertain the persistence of deficits and/or the placement of developmen-tal changes.

SUMMARY

This chapter focused on neuropsychological assessment of the child or adolescent with TBI. It is essential for the pediatric neuropsychologist to examine a number of different areas and to view the results from a developmental perspective. It also is suggested that the clinician work in close correspondence with other professionals—cross-discipline integra-tion is essential to ensure meaningful interpretation of behavior as well as formulation of useful intervention strategies. The role of the neuro-psychological evaluation should be not only to describe functional deficits but also to map strengths and recovery of function.

7

SOCIAL-EMOTIONAL AND BEHAVIORAL ASSESSMENT

An extensive evaluation of children and adolescents who have sustained traumatic brain injury should include a comprehensive appraisal of social-emotional functions. As indicated in Chapter 4, certain subsamples of traumatically brain-injured children and adolescents are at significant risk for behavioral difficulties. These behavioral difficulties can impact upon the adjustment of the child or adolescent back into the home, school, and community environments. The ultimate goal of a comprehensive evaluation of social-emotional functions should be to determine contributory factors from the TBI, as well as to structure an effective intervention program.

The evaluation of social-emotional functions with the child or adolescent with TBI can be a complex process. A number of factors need to be considered, such as the extent of the injury, premorbid functioning, readjustment following a traumatic situation, residual cognitive deficits, and contributory factors such as effects of medication. The experienced clinician needs to review all of these factors to make more accurate diagnostic decisions and subsequent recommendations for treatment. A behaviorally based assessment is thought to yield the most important and useful information and will be the primary focus of this chapter. Such assessment does not preclude the use of other approaches to social-emotional assessment for individuals sustaining a TBI, but neuropsychological findings can impact these methods (e.g., visual-perceptual deficits might distort findings on a Rorschach or Draw-A-Person) and caution should be exercised with their use with individuals with TBI. Regardless of assessment approach, it is critical to account for premorbid social-emotional functioning as well as cognitive factors that can contribute to behavioral deficits. As with other assessments, the social-emotional/behavioral evaluation involves several distinct components.

REVIEW OF
BACKGROUND INFORMATION

As with the comprehensive neuropsychological evaluation, it is critical when evaluating social-emotional and behavioral functions to obtain as much background information as possible. It is important to review all available records to formulate a clear picture of premorbid behavioral functioning. This is particularly relevant for those individuals who have sustained mild-to-moderate injuries as these populations seem to be at less risk for subsequent development of persistent behavioral problems.

The collection of accurate background information is a multistep process that should involve contact with a number of individuals who are familiar with the child or adolescent. Formal interviews with these individuals should focus on gathering information concerning exact behavioral and emotional characteristics of the child or adolescent prior to the accident. When possible, it is always advantageous to validate obtained information through more than one source.

Review of school records also can provide important information, including group test scores as well as any previous individual evaluations that may have been completed in the school environment. Given that TBI does not appear to be randomly distributed, many children or adolescents who sustain a traumatic brain injury may have been previously evaluated or referred for behavioral difficulties. If possible, these reports should be obtained and thoroughly reviewed. The clinician also may want to conduct follow-up interviews with any teachers or clinical professionals who have had contact with the injured individual.

Other important sources of information are medical records. In particular, it is useful to see if the individual has been placed on any psychotropic medications or other types of medicines that may have been used for treatment of behavioral or emotional problems. Other premorbid medical conditions, such as a seizure disorder, that can impact behavior need to be considered in establishing the preinjury social-emotional status of the individual.

Once all pertinent information has been gathered, the clinician should, in most cases, be able to formulate a fairly good pattern of premorbid behavioral and emotional functions. At this point, the clinician is ready to proceed with the formalized assessment of current social and emotional functioning.

ASSESSMENT OF SOCIAL-EMOTIONAL AND BEHAVIORAL STATUS

Behavioral Interview

As mentioned above, interviews with significant others play a primary role in collection of premorbid status information. The interview also plays an important role in the assessment of the child or adolescent's current status. The clinician should initiate this phase by interviewing parents. The focus should be from an informal standpoint to gain parental perspectives concerning changes in the child or adolescent's behavior following the traumatic brain injury. An examination of the nature and quality of parent-child interactions and how these may have changed also is warranted. From a behavioral standpoint, problematic behaviors, antecedent stimuli, and environmental consequences play a crucial role in the diagnosis of behavioral difficulties as well as formulation of behavioral interventions.

To obtain diagnostic information, it may be useful to place children and adolescents and their parents in more structured situations. Forehand and McMahon (1981) present such a structured format that focuses on problematic situations. Patterson and Bank (1986) also have developed a structured parental interview format. These systems focus on a broad range of issues relevant to parenting styles as well as the parent-child interactions. Not only are these types of interviews useful in providing information concerning parent-child interactions and how parents respond to certain situations, but they can be enlightening to parents in regard to their particular style and response to the child or adolescent's behaviors.

Every attempt should be made to interview the teacher of the child or adolescent of concern. The focus should be on collecting information concerning classroom behaviors and interactions of the child or adolescent with the teacher as well as peers. Data should be gathered about appropriate and inappropriate behaviors the child or adolescent demonstrates in the formal classroom setting as well as less structured situations (e.g., lunchroom, recess). It is always useful to interview teachers who may have had the child or adolescent prior to the accident to gain information concerning significant changes in classroom behavior. Furthermore, it is useful to analyze the classroom environment, focusing on rules that are established, behavioral programs that may be in existence, expectations for the child, and teacher-parent communication.

An individual interview with the child or adolescent is important. Although this may not yield reliable information concerning behavioral symptomatology, it does afford the opportunity to gain the individual's perception on his or her functioning pre- and postinjury. Behavioral observations also can be obtained from this interview. Included in the child or adolescent interview should be perceptions of changes in the person's behavior/cognitive abilities, perceptions of adjustments to current situations, satisfaction with provided services, perception of teacher/parent-child or parent-teacher conflicts, and physical symptomatology. In this interview, the clinician can gather observations on sustained attention, appropriateness of verbal responses, impulsiveness, personal insight, and many other qualitative aspects of behavioral functioning. This interview also can be utilized as an opportunity for the clinician to build rapport with the child or adolescent, as this is often the initial stage of a more comprehensive evaluation. Structured interviews also can be a part of any follow-up assessment, allowing the clinician to incorporate and report both objective and subjective information with regard to behavioral changes.

Behavior Checklist

Behavioral rating scales play a key component in psychosocial evaluations of children and adolescents. These scales are usually completed by parents or teachers in reference to a child or adolescent's observable behaviors. These scales provide a good measure of significant others' perceptions of behavioral characteristics. Another advantage of these assessment techniques is that they allow others to focus on important behaviors that may alter perceptions. Behavior rating scales also provide baseline data and information toward formulation of intervention strategies as well as an ongoing opportunity to monitor treatment.

There are many behavior rating scales available to clinicians, but it is recommended that selection be based on psychometric as well as practical considerations. For example, the Child Behavior Checklist (CBCL) (Achenbach, 1991) is one of the stronger and more widely used behavioral scales available to clinicians and subscribes to a multisetting, multirater, multi-instrument design (Martin, Hooper, & Snow, 1986). The parental form of the CBCL is standardized for subjects between the ages of 4 through 18; the Teacher Report Form, for ages 5 through 18; and the Youth Self-Report, for ages 11 through 18. A number of specific scales are yielded by this measure as well as broad-based Internalizing and Externalizing factors. In examining the data yielded by these scales, it is sometimes useful to have parents complete both premorbid and postmorbid profiles to enable the clinician to examine significant behavioral changes that may have occurred following the traumatic brain injury. Interparental comparisons also can provide important clinical information, and it can be useful to conduct follow-up interviews with parents following completion of the scale.

Another set of strong behavior rating scales are the Conners' Rating Scales (Conners, 1990). As with the CBCL, the Conners' scales include measures completed by both parents and teachers. There are two versions of the parent rating scale, one involving completion of 93 items, the other with 48 items. Each item is scored in a similar direction, and both scales yield indices of both internalizing and externalizing type behaviors. All versions of the Conners' Rating Scales also include the Hyperactivity Index, consisting of 10 items that, among other things, are most sensitive to use of medications. The Hyperactivity Index is a quickly scored scale that may be utilized as a screening device or a means of assessing intervention strategies if overt hyperactivity is a presenting problem.

There are a variety of behavior rating scales available to the clinician. Although these may be useful with respect to diagnosis, treatment, and treatment monitoring, care should be exercised in their interpretation of the behavioral manifestations of an individual following a TBI. For example, one might expect to see a heightened number of somatic complaints (e.g., headaches) or thought disorganization in an individual sustaining a severe head injury. Without a significant premorbid history, it would be in error to view these behaviors as exclusively psychosomatic or psychotic-like, given that these behaviors typically can be seen following TBI. It might also be in error to view these behaviors as permanent, traitlike behaviors, particularly if an individual is still in the acute recovery phase. In general, caution should be used prior to making any interpretive conclusions from rating scale information.

Behavioral Observations

Direct observation of behavior can be an important component in establishing and measuring target behaviors. Observation of the child or adolescent in the natural environment allows the clinician to examine the nature and extent of behavioral difficulties, behavioral competencies, and environmental consequences. These observations also help in obtaining more meaningful information concerning parent-child or teacher-child interactions.

Information gathered through interviews as well as behavior checklists often provides clues as to the target behaviors that should be the focus of systematic observation. Once target behaviors have been determined, then the appropriate system of observation can be implemented. For example, it may be that a frequency recording is necessary for a behavior of concern. Another focus of observation can include how a behavior is performed in a particular situation. Duration may be another factor, particularly for studying overt behaviors such as temper tantrums, anger outbursts, or sustained attention to task. The clinician also may be interested in examining latency, measuring the time from presentation of a particular environmental prompt to when the desired response occurs or is initiated. Once a system of observation has been established, the clinician can collect baseline data and subsequently evaluate the effectiveness of intervention strategies.

Although direct behavior observation is a preferred method for collection of important behavioral data, practical limitations are a consideration. Clinicians themselves do not often have the time or opportunity to conduct direct behavioral observations in natural settings. If the clinician does not have a technician available to collect this information systematically, it is often not feasible to conduct direct observations outside of the clinical setting. One option is to train individuals in different environmental settings. In this regard, the clinician serves as a consultant and educates parents or teachers to collect the observational data. The problems associated with this method include difficulties assessing the reliability of observations as well as burdening significant others with extra duties. This can be detrimental in maintaining good rapport and therapeutic relationships with parents or other professionals. On the other hand, many of the behavioral observation systems are not complex, and if the systems allow others to view positive behavior change, this can serve to improve the therapeutic relationship.

Clinicians working in hospitals, schools, and other institutional settings may have the opportunity to complete naturalistic observations, but this may not be feasible for all professionals. Consequently, it may be useful to utilize a structured observation procedure in the office setting. Systems have been developed that allow the clinician to create situations and observe parent-child interactions (e.g., Eyberg & Robinson, 1983; Forehand & McMahon, 1981). These systems place the parent and child in situations and provide the opportunity to observe antecedents and consequences for the child or adolescent's compliance and noncompliance. Methods also have been developed for use in home settings (Patterson, Ray, Shaw, & Cobb, 1969; Wahler, House, & Stambaugh, 1976). These structured coding systems allow for assessment of familial social interactions skills focusing on negative as well as positive behaviors. Although such methods may provide useful information, they are somewhat complex to administer and psychometric properties have not been firmly established.

Paper-and-Pencil Measures

In addition to a comprehensive behavioral assessment, completion of paper-and-pencil measures can yield useful information. They can include such basic scales as the Reynolds Adolescent Depression Scale (Reynolds, 1987), the Reynolds Child Depression Scale (Reynolds, 1989), the Revised Children's Manifest Anxiety Scale (Reynolds & Richmond, 1985), and the State-Trait Anger Expression Inventory (Spielberger, 1981). These measures allow clinicians to obtain self-report and subjective information from the child or adolescent. These measures can point toward factors of concern and suggest areas in need of more comprehensive follow-up evaluations.

For older subjects, the clinician may want to use the Minnesota Multiphasic Personality Inventory—Adolescent (MMPI-A). This comprehensive measure represents a downward extension of the traditional adult personality inventory with basically the same scales. Interested clinicians should consult Archer (1992) for a comprehensive review of this measure. It is suggested that this measure be used, along with any other paper-and-pencil test, to corroborate what is obtained through the comprehensive behavioral assessment. It is strongly suggested that clinicians not rely solely on these measures when assessing the traumatically brain-injured child or adolescent. Interpretation of the MMPI-A as well as other paper-and-pencil measures should be made with caution as little empirical evidence is available for these measures with the traumatically brain-injured child and adolescent. In addition, cognitive and/or reading difficulties may preclude valid use of these assessment techniques with this clinical population.

Communication of Results and Assessment Schedules

Following the initial workup of the child or adolescent with TBI, the clinician should communicate the findings on behavioral/emotional difficulties. Although it seems trite to say the report should be written in terms understandable to all professionals who may come into contact with the child or adolescent, this is especially critical if intervention techniques are to be adequately communicated and implemented. The written report should avoid use of psychological jargon and should describe difficulties in more objective behavioral terms. In other words, it is not merely enough to report that a child may be "acting out" or "depressed-withdrawn." It is advantageous to spell out the exact behaviors that led to these diagnostic conclusions. This is not to argue that the clinician may not want to provide an overall diagnostic interpretation, but more specific behavior descriptions will more effectively communicate the exact problems and needs of the child or adolescent.

Frequency of psychosocial/behavioral assessment for the child or adolescent with TBI is an important consideration. Clearly, more frequent evaluations are needed for severely injured patients as these children and adolescents are at significantly greater risks for behavioral difficulties. In addition, assessment should be ongoing for many of these patients if a specific behavioral treatment intervention is implemented. In this regard, comprehensive behavioral data may be collected for certain children and adolescents in tandem with other types of information, such as neuro-psychological functioning, that may impact on social and emotional status.

The evaluating clinician also should be available as a resource consultant. Although an assessment completed in the office setting may yield important information concerning parent-child interactions or specific behaviors of the child or adolescent, new behavioral and emotional difficulties may emerge as the individual enters different environments. For example, reintegration into the school environment can be difficult. The transition can be particularly difficult if specific accommodations are not implemented immediately. At this point, the clinician can provide expert consultation to professionals working with the child. It also may be necessary to provide supportive counseling services to the child as well as other family members. This ongoing process should help to maintain important relationships that are critical for the adequate adjustment of the individual.

SUMMARY

As noted in Chapter 4, children and adolescents who sustain a traumatic brain injury may be at risk for development of behavioral/emotional difficulties. This chapter outlined a predominantly behavioral approach for assessment of psychosocial functioning. We advocate this approach because we believe this method provides the most objective means of evaluating behavior as well as yielding the useful data with regard to producing effective intervention strategies. It also can be cost effective and time efficient. The process is a multistep procedure, involving structured interviews, behavior ratings, systematic observations, and confirmation of observed difficulties through paper-and-pencil measures. Follow-up evaluations are necessary to track the course of behavior change.

8

INTERVENTION STRATEGIES

Following a comprehensive evaluation an effective intervention plan can be generated. As with any clinical population, specific interventions can play a critical role in the overall recovery process for the child or adolescent with TBI. It is critical that all aspects of functioning be considered when developing a comprehensive treatment plan. In this regard, the clinician or interdisciplinary team needs to focus on the various environments to which the patient will return. This makes it critical to formulate a plan that addresses aspects of behavior in the academic, community, and home environments.

TREATMENT IN
THE SCHOOL ENVIRONMENT

Transition Back to School

Although many children and adolescents with TBI may not be hospitalized, for those who are one of the more critical aspects of treatment is a smooth transition back to the school environment. As the clinician works with school officials, it is important that flexible programming be maintained (Ylvisaker, Hartwick, & Stevens, 1991). During the transition process, school officials need to be informed about the particular strengths and weaknesses of the child. Academic as well as social support should be considered in the transition.

The transition back to school needs to be as smooth as possible. The child may have been away from the home environment for an extended length of time, which in and of itself can be stressful. This traumatic event also can be extremely difficult for family members, and specific treatment to families will be discussed later in the chapter. Many children and adolescents also may have had a less than successful premorbid academic experience. When significant cognitive or emotional deficits secondary to TBI are present, the transition back to what was previously a difficult environment likely will be all the more stressful. The goal, therefore, should be to minimize the anxiety experienced by the individual while maximizing the potential for academic and social success.

A critical factor to be discussed with the school officials is the length of the school day. In many cases, it is not feasible to transition initially to a full school day. Younger children who have sustained moderate-to-severe head injuries may only be able to tolerate a couple of hours a day in the school environment. The professional working with the child or adolescent should be able to recommend the appropriate length of time to spend in the academic environment. Regular consultation with school officials also allows input as to the child's status and provides guidelines for gradually increasing the time in which the child can effectively function in school.

Efforts also should be made to maintain consistency with academic programming. As emphasized by Ylvisaker et al. (1991), it may be useful to obtain academic materials familiar to the child or adolescent prior to his or her return to school. Furthermore, it is important to maintain consistency in the teachers and specialists who may be working with the child or adolescent. If a new group of teachers and other professionals will be working with the child, the clinician should regularly consult with these professionals and provide background information and strategies. Not only should initial contact be made with other professionals, the experienced clinician should be available on a regular basis as a consultant to facilitate any changes that may be needed in the individual's program. This is particularly important as it is strongly recommended that regular follow-up assessments be conducted.

In-service training can be a useful tool in facilitating smooth transitions for children and adolescents with TBI. Studies have indicated that many school professionals lack sufficient knowledge concerning TBI (e.g., Cooley & Singer, 1991). A series of in-services could be presented to familiarize school personnel with the characteristics of children and adolescents with TBI as well as to illustrate specific techniques that may be utilized to deal with this clinical population effectively. At a minimum, it is important that the training emphasize recovery of function, cognitive/behavioral sequelae secondary to traumatic brain injury, emotional factors associated with TBI, behavioral intervention and behavioral management with TBI children and adolescents, and recommended strategies for potential academic interventions. These comprehensive in-services not only provide a forum to communicate information that will ultimately benefit an individual's transition back to the school environment, but also open a doorway to more effective consultative services. It should be made clear to all participants that consultation is available at any point. This may be particularly critical during the early transitional stages.

Recommendations for Placement and Instructional Strategies

As a smooth transition back into the school environment is being facilitated, it becomes necessary to provide recommendations for appropriate academic instruction and placement. Given that a comprehensive evaluation typically includes psychoeducational testing, the clinician can provide recommendations to the school system for services and placement. Services can range from full-time regular education placement to instruction in a self-contained special education classroom.

Savage (1991) discussed several issues in relation to the classification of students as TBI. The first is the medical designation of mild, moderate, or severe and the use of this classification as an indicator of potential outcome. As indicated by Savage (1991), initial severity of a traumatic brain injury may not always be predictive of long-term outcome. Savage (1991) points out a study conducted by the Children's National Medical Center in which preliminary findings showed that many children with mild head injuries did have significant behavioral difficulties whereas some children who had suffered severe head injuries were doing relatively well (Eichelberger & Ball, 1990). This illustrates the importance of regular follow-up assessments for children who have sustained any degree of traumatic brain injury. With regular follow-up assessments providing current cognitive and behavioral information, a clinician is in a better position to consult with the schools concerning placement.

The second issue discussed by Savage (1991) concerned rehabilitative therapies that schools are required to provide. This is a key issue for many school districts as comprehensive rehabilitative services can be expensive. Cost factors aside, recommendations should be based on the needs of the specific child or adolescent. If a wide variety of services is necessary to enhance recovery or restoration or rehabilitation of skills for the child, than these should be recommended. It is then the school district's responsibility to decide what services are educationally relevant, which ones can be provided and ways for paying for the relevant services. A strong liaison relationship with the school can be helpful here in that supportive data for specific recommendations can be provided in a nonconfrontational manner. It also is important that close contact be maintained with other disciplines and that recommendations for treatment be streamlined whenever feasible.

Recommendations for Academic Intervention

Beyond facilitating a smooth transition back into the school environment, as well as providing data helpful toward decision making, it is important to provide recommendations for instructional strategies for the student. These recommendations should be based on data obtained through individual testing, behavioral observation, and therapy sessions. At one level, the clinician may be involved with the development of an individual education plan (IEP). Consultation may be necessary with teachers who are developing this plan as they may not be familiar with TBI. Not all students, however, may qualify for direct special education services. It then may become necessary to provide recommendations and strategies for regular education teachers to facilitate adjustment to the classroom environment. This situation is likely where more exact recommendations for academic instruction are going to be necessary as compared to when the child is placed in special education with a trained special education teacher who can formulate specific strategies.

Glang, Singer, Cooley, and Tish (1992) described what they call direct instruction techniques with students with TBI. These investigators described the features of direct instruction, including the assumption that all students can learn if instruction is presented in a logical, unambiguous, and clear manner. This technique is behavioral in nature and utilizes task analysis, shaping, modeling, and reinforcement. Unique features of the direct instruction model include the following: Skills are pretaught, problem-solving strategies are developed, wording of instructions is consistent, corrections are built into the instructions to provide immediate practice with more difficult tasks, mastery is ensured at each step of the learning process, and a cumulative review of all skills ensures integration with previously learned material. These investigators presented data for three case studies that included an 8-year-old, a 6-year-old, and a 10-year-old. A variety of techniques was illustrated across different subject material. Systematic observations were collected for all three subjects and the results suggested positive increases beyond baseline data. This method thus appears promising, but the investigators also point out limitations. They did not examine the generalization of the results into the classroom setting. Furthermore, it appears as if this technique is best suited for classroom settings with a low teacher-to-student ratio. As Glang et al. (1992) point out, the direct instruction technique takes considerable training. This represents one of the few systematic studies designed to examine effects of various academic inter- vention techniques at facilitating skill development with children with TBI.

Cohen (1991) also presented strategies that may be useful in making recommendations to classroom teachers. As indicated, there are differing goals that may be established for the child or adolescent during early, middle, and later stages of the recovery process following a traumatic brain injury. This calls for the need for continuous follow-up and the close documentation of progress and skill acquisition. Cohen (1991) points out a number of strategies that may be utilized with these students, noting that these students should be placed in active learning situations and should learn through participation. This requires some flexibility on the part of the teacher, as well as active and close feedback contingencies. Cohen (1991) also indicated the need to evaluate the complexity of task presentation closely and to present material at an appropriate pace. In addition, the teacher needs to focus on specific student characteristics such as derived from neuropsychological (e.g., impulsivity, memory) and psychosocial (e.g., depression) evaluations.

A third factor addressed by Cohen (1991) is the need to deal with specific deficits as well as provide instructions for skill development. Cohen (1991) suggested that generalized problems, such as attention difficulties, decreased comprehension, dysfunctional organization skills, or memory deficits can have devastating affects on the child's acquisition of new information. Calling for specific strategies to address these generalized problems, Cohen (1991) goes on to point out the need to teach the process of an activity and to develop problem-solving strategies. This, again, dictates close monitoring on the part of the teacher, and appropriate contingencies of reinforcement to ensure that the student is using appropriate problem-solving strategies. As the child progresses and evidences recovery of function, the need arises to develop and foster further independence. As the teacher develops particular skills with the child, he or she may be able to reduce some of the monitoring and educational strategies in a systematic fashion and allow the student to utilize new found skills more independently.

The last area addressed by Cohen (1991) is generalization of instruction, including teaching strategies to allow the student to develop appropriate problem-solving skills in different situations. These should facilitate adjustment in the school environment as well as other settings.

TREATMENT SERVICES
TO THE FAMILY

Beyond consulting with school districts, a critical factor in a child's adjustment is the availability of services to both the child and the family. Provision of services can be difficult in that the home and community environments may be less structured than a school setting. In most cases, closer monitoring and more intense intervention on the part of the clinician will be necessary.

In relation to the family situation, it is important to establish baseline data as to the premorbid functioning level. Through systematic interviews and other sources of information, it may become clear that dysfunction was present in the family system prior to the onset of the traumatic injury. Such a situation may be further compounded by the factors relating to family adjustment following the traumatic condition, as well as adjustment of significant others to changes in the individual. In general, numerous factors must be considered when designing specific interventions to the family. The clinician needs to consider both premorbid conditions and adaptation to the current situation. There are numerous behavioral and psychosocial interventions available (see Kazdin, 1988), and discussion of specific techniques is beyond the scope of this volume. The factors that should be considered in the selection of intervention techniques include:

1. Family issues—Is there a need for family systems intervention? If so, are the issues to be addressed specific to current situations surrounding the injured patient? Are there also premorbid factors that need to be considered?

2. Developmental issues, including the current developmental status of the child or adolescent and projections as to what the implications of the traumatic brain injury may be on future developmental progress.

3. Specific environment and individual differences relevant to formulating a treatment plan.

4. Efficiency and ease with which a specific intervention program can be implemented, monitored, and changed.

5. Frequency and intensity of intervention strategies.

6. Involvement of family members as well as significant others within the therapeutic modality.

7. Consultation with other professionals outside of the therapeutic situation to maintain generalization of intervention strategies.

8. Monitoring and documentation of specific outcomes.

Individual psychotherapy services also may be needed for the child or adolescent with TBI. Readers interested in an excellent overview of psychotherapy with children and adolescents are directed to Kazdin (1993); however, very little research is available concerning psychotherapy interventions in a pediatric TBI population. In general terms, the overall goals of psychotherapy with this population should be the same as with any other clinical population. These goals should include decreasing maladaptive or inappropriate behaviors and increasing appropriate prosocial behaviors. Specific psychotherapy should enable the child or adolescent to become more adaptable to changing environments. The specific technique utilized should depend on the presenting problem as well as other issues. It is critical that the therapist providing the psychotherapy have a thorough understanding of not only the behavioral/emotional characteristics of the child or adolescent but also the cognitive factors. For example, engaging in a talking therapy with an individual showing language residuals from a TBI may not be efficient in accomplishing behavioral change.

The design of a psychotherapeutic intervention program can be a complex process with the brain-injured child or adolescent. As noted in earlier chapters, the pattern for the child or adolescent with TBI can be quite dynamic as recovery of function progresses. This calls for flexibility with the type of intervention implemented. Furthermore, cognitive factors need to be considered when dealing with this clinical population. From one standpoint, it is important to determine the extent to which cognitive deficits in different environments are contributing to the emotional or behavioral problems evidenced by the child or adolescent. It might be useful to incorporate cognitive training techniques as thinking skill deficits may be the primary underlying etiology of maladaptive behavioral patterns. It also is important for the therapist to consider the cognitive deficits when utilizing therapeutic techniques. Cognitive limitations may have a direct impact on use of insight-oriented therapies or techniques that load heavily on problem solving, mental flexibility, and memory. Yet another factor that needs to be considered is the extent to which consultation with other professionals is necessary throughout the process. The therapist may want to institute programs that are easily implemented in the school environment. Consequently, it will be necessary to consult closely with school officials and continue to advocate for adequate training and delivery of therapeutic intervention strategies.

Finally, as with any intervention technique, it is absolutely critical to monitor the progress being made by the child or adolescent, preferably from an empirical perspective. This allows the opportunity to make needed changes as well as to maintain close contact with parents, teachers, and other professionals.

SUMMARY

Specific intervention techniques are extremely important in facilitating the readjustment of the child or adolescent with TBI to communities outside of a hospital or rehabilitation environment. The reintegration of these individuals can pose significant challenges. One of the primary settings is the school environment. It is absolutely critical that professionals consult with school officials to facilitate a smooth transition back to this challenging environment. In addition, specific treatment of both family and individual often is necessary. The degree to which a successful intervention strategy is implemented can have long-term effects on the development and eventual adjustment of the child or adolescent. The ultimate goal is to foster as much independence as possible, given the presence of specific cognitive and emotional/behavioral deficits. This smooth transition and development is best accomplished through an interdisciplinary team approach with ample monitoring points provided throughout the recovery and developmental processes.

9

ILLUSTRATIVE CASE STUDY

To more clearly illustrate factors discussed in the preceding chapters, we present a case study. Included in this discussion is a review of specific test results. Because of space limitations, detailed descriptions of the measures will not be presented. Readers interested in learning more about these and other neuropsychological assessment techniques are referred to Lezak (1983) and Spreen and Strauss (1991).

The case concerns a 9-year-old boy who will be called G. W. This child was involved in a motor vehicle accident and suffered a severe traumatic brain injury. Upon admission to the emergency room, he had a large laceration on his scalp and a left nystagmus. His left pupil was approximately 3 mm and sluggish; his right pupil was nonreactive. He was reported to have a Glasgow Coma Scale of approximately 4. The child underwent an emergency craniotomy for elevation of a depressed skull fracture and debridement of the left frontal lobe. He subsequently underwent open reduction/internal fixation of nasal and frontal fractures with repair of spinal leaks via a frontal craniotomy. His hospital stay was lengthy, and he received rehabilitative services both as an inpatient and an outpatient.

During his acute hospital stay, G. W. had regular CT scans. Table 9.1 summarizes the results of these studies. The initial scan clearly demonstrated the fractures in the cranial vault as well as hemorrhagic contusions. Subsequent studies continued to show the right frontal hemorrhagic contusion as well as a midline shift. His neuroanatomical status changed as time progressed. Resolution was noted of the hemorrhagic contusion with less persistent midline shift. As swelling and shifts decreased, it should be noted there was an enlargement of this child's lateral ventricles, which probably represents early cerebral atrophy. Also noted was progressive encephalomalacia.

TABLE 9.1 Serial CT Scans and Changing Results

Study #	Impression/Results
1	Shows fractures in both the orbital roof and superior orbital rim. A fracture is also noted in the cranial vault in the left frontal and parietal regions with a depressed fragment measuring approximately 7 cm in length. A possible fracture was also noted in the floor of the left anterior cranial fossa. Hemorrhagic contusions are noted in the frontal lobe regions with surrounding edema. A small amount of blood was noted in the occipital horn of the left lateral ventricle.
2	The frontal hemorrhagic contusions were relatively stable from the previous study. There was no evidence of any new hemorrhaging. A midline shift is noted in this study. There continues to be blood in the posterior aspect of the left lateral ventricle and occipital horn.
3	Decreased mass affect is noted in the temporal, frontal, and occipital horns of the right lateral ventricle. The frontal hemorrhagic contusions remain relatively stable. There was a slight decrease noted in the amount of the midline shift.
4	This study began to show resolution of the hypodense lesions in the frontal areas. There was continued decreased effacement in the frontal horn of the right lateral ventricle. This study showed the midline shift to be minimal. There continued to be blood in the posterior region of the left lateral ventricle.
5	This study noted continued resolution of hypodensities in the frontal areas. Mild enlargement of the lateral ventricles is noted in this scan, which is suggestive of early cerebral atrophy. No new evidence of acute hemorrhages is noted and the midline shift continued to be minimal.
6	This study noted continued resolution of the contusions in the bi-frontal areas. Areas of decreased attenuation are noted, which is consistent with progressive encephalomalacia. No new hemorrhages were noted. These studies continue to show enlargement of the lateral ventricles.

This case study illustrates the effectiveness and importance of serial CT scanning. Early scans demonstrated acute conditions critical to medical monitoring, including the contusions and the midline shift. As these factors resolved, more long-standing deficits became evident. This is frequently seen in children and adolescents with severe TBI. For this child, there is suggestion of cerebral atrophy as well as encephalomalacia.

This child also had a series of EEG studies with abnormal results. These studies were suggestive of potential seizure focus, and seizure activity was believed to be observed with G. W. Given these factors, he was initially placed on phenobarbital and subsequently switched to Tegretol for seizure control.

NEUROPSYCHOLOGICAL TESTING

As discussed above, serial CT scanning showed initial hemorrhagic contusions in the frontal area with subsequent indications of cerebral atrophy as well as encephalomalacia. In this section, we review background information as well as comprehensive neuropsychological evaluation results.

Background Information

With regard to other medical history, G. W. sustained viral pneumonia at approximately 4 weeks of age. He was hospitalized for a 4- to 5-day period. G. W. had early ear infections, although no tubes were inserted. His hearing was within normal limits. G. W. had no significant premorbid history of neurological difficulties.

G. W.'s mother was approximately 21 years old when she became pregnant. She maintained regular doctor visits. The delivery occurred at approximately 7½ months and was vaginal. G. W.'s birth weight was approximately 5 pounds 15 ounces. He sustained a broken collarbone and his lungs were not well developed. He also showed signs of severe jaundice. G. W. required a 10-day hospital stay, although this was in a regular care nursery. Based on parental report, G. W.'s developmental milestones were within normal limits. He crawled independently at 6 months of age and walked independently at 9 months of age. He was able to ride a bicycle at approximately 4 years of age. He began using single words at approximately 6 months and was able to combine words into meaningful sentences at 2 years. G. W. did not experience significant difficulties with toilet training, although bed-wetting continued to be a persistent problem for this child. G. W. was bottle-fed and showed good sleep patterns throughout infancy.

At the time of the accident, G. W. was enrolled in a regular education second-grade classroom. He had not been retained at any grade level nor was he receiving any special education services prior to the accident. His parents indicated that G. W. was a good student, earning mostly As and Bs.

Family background for this child was relatively unremarkable. G. W. was living with his parents and two siblings at the time of the accident. There was no family history of neurological or learning difficulties. G. W.'s siblings were both healthy with no developmental or academic problems.

G. W. was given a complete neuropsychological and speech/language evaluation approximately 6 months following the accident. Results of testing at that time showed his overall intellectual abilities to be in the average to low average range, although his Verbal Scale IQ was significantly higher than his Performance Scale IQ. Strengths noted from the evaluation included verbal intelligence, verbal memory, and incidental memory for written material. Weaknesses were found in the areas of nonverbal perceptual organization abilities, concentration, attention, selective attention, and incidental memory. A relative weakness also was noted in his expressive language functions. Results of the speech/language evaluation showed G. W.'s visual-motor integration skills to be in the borderline range. Psycholinguistic functions were generally depressed, although one-word receptive vocabulary skills and one-word expressive vocabulary abilities were within normal limits. Academic achievement skills were in the borderline to low average range.

Psychoeducational Evaluation

Table 9.2 lists scores for the psychoeducational evaluation completed with G. W. In examining this table, it can be seen that his overall intellectual skills are well within the average range. G. W. did not evidence a significant split between his Verbal and Performance scales, suggesting relatively even development of intellectual abilities. He did demonstrate some variability among his subtests. G. W. appears to have problems on tests that tap attention and concentration. A relative strength is noted in the area of social intelligence.

With regard to academic skills, G. W. also shows considerable variability. His reading skills appear to be within the average to high average range. G. W. demonstrates a particular strength in the area of reading comprehension. His math skills appear to be somewhat more problematic. G. W. is particularly low in basic math calculation abilities. Another area of extreme deficit is in written expression: G. W. had difficulties on a subtest requiring generation of sentences.

TABLE 9.2 Psychoeducational Summary

Test	Score
WISC-R	
Information	6
Similarities	11
Arithmetic	7
Vocabulary	11
Comprehension	15
Picture Completion	7
Picture Arrangement	12
Block Design	11
Object Assembly	12
Coding	8
Verbal Scale IQ	100
Performance Scale IQ	100
Full Scale IQ	100
Woodcock-Johnson Revised	
Letter/Word Identification	94
Passage Comprehension	105
Calculations	77
Applied Problems	85
Dictation	78
Writing Samples	52

Motor, Sensory, and Perceptual Scores

Table 9.3 lists scores on a number of different measures. In psychomotor performance, G. W. evidenced a slight left-hand advantage. This is problematic as G. W. is right-hand dominant. His strength, however, was in the predicted direction. G. W.'s overall abilities in these areas are not highly suggestive of significant psychomotor slowing or decreased strength.

Tactile integration abilities appear to be extremely problematic for this child. He evidenced bilateral depression on both the Tactile Finger Recognition Test as well as the Fingertip Number Writing Test. These results would indicate possible bilateral dysfunction with regard to tactile integration abilities.

Visual-perceptual abilities also were assessed using a number of different measures. His performance on Part A of the Trail Making Test was within

TABLE 9.3 Motor, Sensory, and Perceptual Scores

Test	Score
Finger Tapping	R=34.9, L=36
Grip Strength	R=18, L=16
Tactile Finger Recognition	R=7 errors, L=6 errors
Fingertip Number Writing	R=14 errors, L=15 errors
Trail Making Test, Part A	28 seconds
Visual Form Discrimination	Total Correct: 26
Line Orientation	Total Correct: 14
Facial Recognition Test	Total Correct: 37
Bender-Gestalt	Developmental Errors: 8

normal limits. This would indicate intact visual scanning and visual sequencing skills. He did show a slight depression with regard to visual matching ability, although he was somewhat impulsive in responding on this measure. Visual-spatial orientation abilities are depressed, as are facial recognition skills.

G. W. committed a number of developmental errors on a measure of visual-motor integration, suggesting significant delay and/or dysfunction. His errors were of different types, including distortions, integration problems, and perseverations.

Memory Functions

Table 9.4 lists scores on memory testing for G. W. These results indicate difficulties with memory functions. His overall memory abilities appear to be in the mildly deficient to borderline range. G. W. is particularly low in the area of visual memory. Although verbal memory is a relative strength for this child, it is still well below what would be expected given his average level of intellectual functioning. The overall pattern suggests deficits with encoding/consolidation as well as consistent retrieval. These findings are further supported by his performance on the Selective Reminding Test. Although G. W. does appear able to retain some information in short-term memory and has the ability to transfer information into long-term storage, he is particularly deficient in his consistent retrieval of information from long-term storage.

TABLE 9.4 Memory Functions

Test	Score
Wide Range Assessment of Memory and Learning	
Picture Memory	9
Design Memory	2
Verbal Learning	6
Story Memory	9
Finger Windows	3
Sound Symbol	6
Sentence Memory	8
Visual Learning	5
Number/Letter	4
Verbal Memory Index	81
Visual Memory Index	63
Learning Index	71
General Memory Index	65
Selective Reminding	
Total Recall	45
Long Term Storage	48
Long Term Retrieval	36
Consistent Long Term Retrieval	9

Executive Functions and Attention

G. W.'s performance on Part B of the Trail Making Test was in the severely dysfunctional range. This would indicate difficulties with mental flexibility as well as speeded mental processing. His performance on the Wisconsin Card Sorting Test also was problematic. He was only able to complete four categories correctly and he showed 47 perseverative responses. G. W. also had one failure to maintain set. These overall results suggest that he has difficulty utilizing limited environmental feedback to facilitate problem solving, a perseverative response style, and potential attention difficulties while engaged in higher cognitive tasks (see Table 9.5).

Attention/vigilance and impulsive responding were assessed using the Continuous Performance Test. The overall results on this measure were well below what would be expected for a child of his age and demonstrated intellectual abilities. The low absolute percent correct score suggests that G. W. has difficulties with sustained visual attention. The depressed relative percent score suggests impulsivity in giving responses.

TABLE 9.5 Executive Functions

Test	Score
Trail Making Test, Part B	218 seconds
Wisconsin Card Sort Test	
Categories Completed	4
Perseverative Responses	47
Perseverative Errors	39
Failure to Maintain Set	1
Continuous Performance Test	
Absolute Percentage Correct	74.0
Relative Percentage Correct	75.51

Summary and Integration

The results of this neuropsychological evaluation point toward a number of specific cognitive weaknesses for G. W. He has shown some recovery of function with general intellectual abilities. G. W. was somewhat impulsive in giving responses and was occasionally distracted by external stimuli. His academic profile suggests reading skills to be within average limits. G. W. shows mild-to-moderate deficits in the area of mathematics and a significant difficulty with written output. Remote memory and retrieval of previously learned material appears to be intact, although G. W. shows significant deficits in the area of recent memory and new learning. Motor functions appear to be generally intact, although G. W. does show a left-hand advantage with regard to psychomotor speed. Tactile integration is depressed bilaterally. G. W. shows difficulties with abstraction and problem-solving abilities and evidences a perseverative response style. G. W. also has difficulties with sustained attention and vigilance and is impulsive in giving responses.

The overall neuropsychological pattern for this child is consistent with what would be expected given his severe traumatic brain injury. He is demonstrating recovery of function with regard to certain skills, particularly verbal comprehension abilities and remote memory skills. He continues to evidence a number of specific deficits that relate primarily to difficulties with recent memory and new learning, speeded mental processing, and depressed executive functions. This profile is not only consistent with generalized deficits often associated with severe TBI, but the more specific damage for G. W., which is in the bifrontal areas.

BEHAVIORAL/
SOCIAL-EMOTIONAL EVALUATION

Behavioral Observations

G. W. was observed during individual testing. His behavior was generally appropriate, although he did appear to be mildly impulsive in giving responses. G. W. did not show overt frustration secondary to failure on more difficult items. He appeared to put forth good effort on the various tasks. Although he did not present with severe signs suggestive of significant attention difficulties, G. W. did tend to be easily distracted by external stimuli. He would return to task with a simple verbal or visual prompt. G. W. responded well to positive verbal feedback. His affect was appropriate throughout the testing and he did not demonstrate any bizarre behaviors.

Table 9.6 summarizes results for behavior ratings. Two of G. W.'s current teachers as well as his parents completed the scales. In examining the profile for the teachers, G. W. does tend to present with externalizing type difficulties. The ratings for the two teachers are very similar. Both rated G. W. significantly high in the areas of hyperactivity, conduct problems, and emotionality.

G. W.'s parents were asked to complete behavior ratings as to his current functions as well as to provide an estimate of his behavior prior to the accident. This was done as an attempt to establish the presence of any premorbid behavior difficulties. Both the mother and father's preaccident ratings profiles are within normal limits. His parents completed these ratings separately, and there is a high correspondence between how he was rated by both his mother and father. In the parent postinjury ratings, there are significant elevations on Conduct Disorder, Restless-Disorganized, Psychosomatic, and Hyperactive-Immature. Again, these results are consistent in indicating externalizing type difficulties.

To briefly summarize, G. W. presents with behavior problems in both the home and school setting. Based on premorbid parental ratings, it does not appear that he had any significant difficulties prior to his severe traumatic brain injury. His ratings across the different environments are consistent, suggesting externalizing difficulties. These social-emotional difficulties can be attributed to a number of factors, including decreased cognitive functions, residual damage to specific cortical and subcortical areas, and emotional adjustment difficulties secondary to the traumatic incident.

TABLE 9.6 Summary of Behavior Rating Scale Profiles

Teacher Rating	Teacher 1	Teacher 2
Hyperactivity	79	74
Conduct	75	75
Emotional	77	77
Anxious-Passive	66	63
Asocial	60	60
Day Dream-Attn.	60	51
Hyperactivity Index	80	75

	Mother		Father	
Parent Ratings	Before	After	Before	After
Conduct Disorder	42	74	49	67
Anxious-Shy	56	61	58	65
Restless-Disorganized	46	84	54	80
Learning Problem	46	57	43	54
Psychosomatic	41	71	51	74
Obsessive-Compulsive	47	52	47	57
Anti-Social	43	53	48	53
Hyperactive-Immature	50	68	52	63

INTERVENTION
RECOMMENDATIONS

In summary, results of neurodiagnostic studies showed initial frontal hemorrhagic contusions with subsequent indications of cerebral atrophy and increasing encephalomalacia. This points toward specific structural/anatomical residual damage for this child. The neuropsychological evaluation was also problematic and was consistent with severe TBI as well as residual damage located predominantly in the frontal regions. G. W. has shown good recovery of function of his general intellectual abilities and well as his remote memory skills. He continues to show significant problems with recent memory abilities, sustained attention/concentration, problem solving, and visual-motor integration. With academic functions, G. W. demonstrates deficits on tasks requiring organization and output. This is particularly the case with his written skills. Social-emotional testing was consistent across both the school and home environments. In general, it appears that G. W. did not have any significant behavioral difficulties premorbidly. His postinjury profile is suggestive of a child with externalizing type problems, including hyperactivity, difficulties with focused attention, and impulsivity. The evaluation suggests the need for a comprehensive intervention strategy for this child. In general, the following recommendations appear to be warranted:

1. G. W. continues to need adjustments in of his transition back to the school environment. The majority of his academic instruction will be provided in the special education classroom, although it is imperative that all of G. W.'s teachers stay in close communication and provide consistent programming. Specific strategies that need to be developed in the school environment include compensatory methods for dealing with difficulties with memory and new learning. In particular, this would be the case for material presented visually. Any teachers working with G. W. will need to present directions either verbally, or keep them visible and short. It may be necessary to repeat directions frequently to allow G. W. the opportunity to encode the information.

2. G. W. continues to show difficulties with executive processes, including a moderate-to-severe deficit with mental flexibility. This places him at risk for making smooth transitions from one task to another. A possible recommendation in this area would be to encourage teachers to be aware of this problem and to allow G. W. some "warm-up" time when he is expected to engage in a new activity. It is also important for teachers to monitor G. W.'s performance on various tasks and provide him with subtle cuing to facilitate necessary shifts within and between tasks.

3. G. W. shows problems with organization and output skills. He will need a structured environment as well as strategies to facilitate organization and planning. Such strategies can include training in specific outlining skills as well as use of a memory log. Other external organizers, such as outlines of daily activities, also would be useful.

4. G. W. continues to show problems with visual-motor integration and visual-motor output. This can have a direct impact on his handwriting abilities, among others. It may be recommended to teachers that G. W. not be graded for penmanship. It also may be useful to allow this child to dictate written assignments. Given his difficulties with speeded motor output as

well as his extreme dysfunction in visual memory, G. W. also should not be required to engage in lengthy copying tasks. As he moves up in grades, it will be important to monitor G. W.'s note-taking abilities. If he does not show considerable recovery of function with a number of skills, this will be a difficult area for him. One possible solution would be to allow G. W. to tape-record lecture material. This would provide him the opportunity to go back and listen to lectures and fill in any gaps he may have in his written notes.

5. The results of both the neuropsychological and social-emotional evaluations point toward externalizing type difficulties for this child. One recommendation would be to create a specific behavior management program for G. W. The focus of this program should be to increase sustained attention to complete assignments as well as focus on improvements in the quality of output. This program should be created in conjunction with G. W.'s parents as well as his teachers to ensure consistency across different environments and increase the effectiveness of the program.

6. In meetings, G. W.'s parents indicated a number of concerns about their family situation. G. W.'s mother was currently seeking individual counseling for treatment of acute depression. G. W.'s older sibling also was beginning to experience behavior difficulties in both school and at home. Given the significant trauma and stress to which this family was subjected, a recommendation should be made for family counseling. Furthermore, G. W.'s parents should receive parent training to manage his behavior more effectively as well as improve the quality of their interactions with him and their other children.

7. Given that G. W. sustained a severe TBI, he should be reevaluated in approximately one year. This would allow the examiner to monitor his cognitive recovery of function closely as well as continue to pinpoint areas of deficit.

These recommendations are only a few of many that could be made for G. W. Clearly, an interdisciplinary approach is going to be needed for this child to address the breadth of his difficulties. Specific academic recommendations could continue to evolve as teachers become more familiar with his strengths and weaknesses. Interdisciplinary communication would be critical for effective programming.

SUMMARY

This chapter presents data and discussion for a 9-year-old boy who sustained a severe TBI. His profile and residual deficits are representative of this clinical population as well as the residual damage secondary to the injury. As can be seen, considerable effort is needed to provide an adequate assessment of this child's cognitive and behavioral functions. Follow-up will be essential to facilitating maximum recovery for this child. This demands a significant commitment on the part of the evaluating clinician.

This case study presents just a few of the issues that need to considered when working with children and adolescents with TBI. The complexities of this clinical population have been illustrated in the preceding chapters. As with any group, research results provide general guidelines that allow formulation of more effective assessment and intervention strategies. Clinicians need to focus on the unique qualities of each child or adolescent referred. Consider what has been presented in this volume as a general framework or foundation for working with children and adolescents with TBI.

Part IV

Postscript

POSTSCRIPT

As mentioned in the preface, this volume was designed to be an introductory overview of traumatic brain injury in children and adolescents. Great strides have been achieved in this area in the last two decades. Research has provided insight as to the recovery of various cognitive and behavioral processes. Residual deficits in these areas also have been examined in a systematic fashion. In spite of the accumulated knowledge, it seems that we are just at the beginning of truly understanding this complex clinical population, and several key issues continue to confront this field.

First, the way in which TBI disrupts the developmental process needs to be more thoroughly examined. Although we do have some understanding as to the course that recovery of function frequently follows, longitudinal studies are needed to examine effects on emerging skills and how qualitative shifts from one stage to another may be impaired. Along these lines, following children and adolescents into adulthood is another area of needed study. For example, Satz (1993) suggested that brain injury may make individuals more susceptible to other neurological disorders, particularly dementing disorders, as these traumatic events can reduce the individual's brain reserve capacity. Such questions hold great promise for increasing our knowledge of the long-term impact of TBI.

Second, techniques in the area of imaging and brain activity continue to advance at a remarkable pace. With this ever-increasing technology, it should become possible to track the neurophysiological aspects of TBI more accurately and to come to a more precise understanding of the relationship between anatomical substrates and cognitive/behavioral correlates. This should increase our effectiveness in predicting functional outcomes as well as designing effective intervention strategies.

Third, systematic investigations are needed to examine intervention strategies with pediatric TBI populations. Variables such as severity of injury, premorbid status, educational placement, and many others need to be controlled and examined in the context of what are critical factors to consider in designing an intervention program. Studies are also needed to investigate the effectiveness of various techniques in bringing about positive behavior change. Family adjustment and parent training are other issues that need to be addressed with respect to TBI.

Through the combined efforts of professionals, knowledge concerning TBI with children and adolescents should continue to increase at a remarkable pace. This will result in more systematic developmental theories as well as strategies to maximize potential with TBI victims. It is our hope that this volume has contributed to these efforts.

REFERENCES

Achenbach, T. M. (1991). *An integrative guide for the 1991 CBCL/4-18, YSR, and TRF Profiles.* Burlington: University of Vermont, Department of Psychiatry.

Adams, J. H., Graham, D. I., & Gennarelli, T. A. (1985). Contemporary neuropathological considerations regarding brain damage in head injury. In D. P. Becker & J. T. Povlishock (Eds.), *Central nervous system trauma status report—1985.* Washington, DC: National Institute for Neurological and Communicative Disorders and Stroke, National Institutes of Health.

Aicardi, J. (1987). *Epilepsy in children.* New York: Raven Press.

Alexander, R. C., Schor, D. P., & Smith, W. L., Jr. (1986). Magnetic resonance imaging of intracranial injuries from child abuse. *Journal of Pediatrics, 109,* 975-979.

Annegers, J. F. (1983). The epidemiology of head trauma in children. In K. Shapiro (Ed.), *Pediatric head trauma* (pp. 1-10). Mount Kisco, NY: Futura.

Annegers, J. F., Grabow, J. D., Kurland, L. T., & Laws, E. R., Jr. (1980). The incidence, causes, and secular trends of head trauma in Olmsted County, Minnesota, 1935-1974. *Neurology, 30,* 912-919.

Archer, R. P. (1992). *MMPI-A: Assessing adolescent psychopathology.* Hillsdale, NJ: Lawrence Erlbaum.

Auerbach, S. H. (1986). Neuroanatomical correlates of attention and memory disorders in traumatic brain injury: An application of neurobehavioral subtypes. *Journal of Head Trauma Rehabilitation, 1,* 1-12.

Bakay, L., & Glasauer, F. E. (1980). *Head injury.* Boston: Little, Brown.

Barona, A., Reynolds, C. R., & Chastain, R. (1984). A demographically based index of pre-morbid intelligence for the WAIS-R. *Journal of Consulting and Clinical Psychology, 52,* 885-887.

Bassett, S. S., & Slater, E. J. (1990). Neuropsychological function in adolescents sustaining mild closed head injury. *Journal of Pediatric Psychology, 15,* 225-236.

Bawden, H. N., Knights, R. M., & Winogron, H. W. (1985). Speeded performance following head injury in children. *Journal of Clinical and Experimental Neuropsychology, 7,* 39-54.

Bennett-Levy, J., & Stores, G. (1984). The nature of cognitive dysfunction in school-children with epilepsy. *Acta Neurologica Scandinavica, 69,* 79-82.

Berger-Gross, P., & Shackelford, M. (1985). Closed head injury in children: Neuropsychological and scholastic outcomes. *Perceptual and Motor Skills, 61,* 254.

115

Bigler, E. D. (1990). Neuropathology of traumatic brain injury. In E. D. Bigler (Ed.), *Traumatic brain injury: Mechanisms of damage, assessment, intervention, and outcome* (pp. 13-49). Austin, TX: Pro-Ed.

Bigler, E. D. (in press). Advances in brain imaging with children and adolescents. In M. G. Tramontana, & S. R. Hooper (Eds.), *Advances in child neuropsychology* (Vol. 3). New York: Springer-Verlag.

Black, P., Jeffries, J., Blumer, D., Wellner, A., & Walker, A. E. (1969). The post-traumatic syndrome in children: Characteristics and incidence. In A. E. Walker, W. F. Caveness, & M. Critchley (Eds.), *The late effects of head injury* (pp. 142-149). Springfield, IL: Charles C Thomas.

Boll, T. J. (1983). Minor head injury in children—Out of sight but not out of mind. *Journal of Clinical Child Psychology, 12,* 74-80.

Bond, M. R. (1983). Effects on the family system. In M. Rosenthal, E. R. Griffith, M. R. Bond, & J. D. Miller (Eds.), *Rehabilitation of the head injured adult* (pp. 209-217). Philadelphia: F. A. Davis.

Brant-Zawadzki, M., & Norman, D. (1987). *Magnetic resonance imaging of the central nervous system.* New York: Raven.

Brink, J. D., Garrett, A. L., Hale, W. R., Woo-Sam, J., & Nickel, V. L. (1970). Recovery of motor and intellectual function in children sustaining severe head injuries. *Developmental Medicine and Child Neurology, 12,* 565-571.

Brodal, A. (1981). *Neurological anatomy in relation to clinical medicine* (3rd ed.). New York: Oxford University Press.

Brooks, D. N. (1983). Disorders of memory. In M. Rosenthal, E. R. Griffith, M. R. Bond, & J. D. Miller (Eds.), *Rehabilitation of the head injured adult* (pp. 185-196). Philadelphia: F. A. Davis.

Brown, G., Chadwick, O., Shaffer, D., Rutter, M., & Traub, M. (1981). A prospective study of children with head injuries: III. Psychiatric sequelae. *Psychological Medicine, 11,* 63-78.

Bruce, D. A., Schut, L., Bruno, L. A., Wood, J. H., & Sutton, L. N. (1978). Outcome following severe head injury in children. *Journal of Neurosurgery, 48,* 679-688.

Bruce, D. A., & Zimmerman, R. A. (1989). Shaken impact syndrome. *Pediatric Annals, 18,* 492-494.

Bucci, M. N., Phillips, T. W., & McGillicuddy, J. E. (1986). Delayed epidural hemorrhage in hypotensive multiple trauma patients. *Neurosurgery, 19,* 65-68.

Burkinshaw, J. (1960). Head injuries in children: Observations on their incidence and causes with an enquiry into the value of routine skull X-rays. *Archives of the Diseases of Children, 35,* 205-214.

Caffey, J. (1974). The whiplash shaken infant syndrome: Manual shaking by the extremities with whiplash-induced intracranial and intraocular bleedings, linked with residual permanent brain damage and mental retardation. *Pediatrics, 54,* 396-403.

Calanchini, P. R., & Trout, S. S. (1971). The neurology of learning disabilities. In L. Tarnopol (Ed.), *Learning disorders in children, diagnosis, medication, education* (pp. 207-251). Boston: Little, Brown.

Casey, R., Ludwig, S., & McCormick, M. (1986). Morbidity following minor head trauma in children. *Pediatrics, 73,* 497-502.

Chadwick, O., Rutter, M., Brown, G., Shaffer, D., & Traub, M. (1981). A prospective study of children with head injuries: II. Cognitive sequelae. *Psychological Medicine, 11,* 49-61.

Chadwick, O., Rutter, M., Shaffer, D., & Shrout, P. E. (1981). A prospective study of children with head injuries: IV. Specific cognitive deficits. *Journal of Clinical Neuropsychology, 3,* 101-120.

Christoffel, K. K. (1990). Violent death and injury in U. S. children and adolescents. *American Journal of Diseases of Children, 144,* 697-706.

Cohen, S. B. (1991). Adapting educational programs for students with head injuries. *Journal of Head Trauma Rehabilitation, 6,* 56-63.

Comninos, S. C. (1979). Early prognosis of severe head injuries in children. *Acta Neurochirurgica, 28,* 144-147.

Conners, C. K. (1990). *Conners' rating scales manual.* North Tonawanda, NY: Multi-Health Systems.

Cooley, E., & Singer, G. (1991). On serving students with head injuries: Are we reinventing a wheel that doesn't roll? *Journal of Head Trauma Rehabilitation, 6,* 47-55.

Cooper, K. D., Tabaddor, K., Hauser, W. A., Schulman, K., Feiner, C., & Factor, P. R. (1983). The epidemiology of head injury in the Bronx. *Neuroepidemiology, 2,* 70-88.

Cooper, P. R. (1982). Epidemiology of head injury. In P. R. Cooper (Ed.), *Head injury* (pp. 1-14). Baltimore, MD: Williams & Wilkins.

Cooper, P. R., Maravilla, K., & Moody, S. (1979). Serial computerized tomographic scanning and the prognosis of severe head injury. *Neurosurgery, 5,* 566-569.

Corbett, M. B., & Trimble, M. R. (1983). Epilepsy and anticonvulsant medication. In M. Rutter (Ed.), *Developmental neuropsychiatry* (pp. 112-129). New York: Guilford.

Courjon, J. (1972). Traumatic disorders. In A. Redmond (Ed.), *Handbook of electroencephalography and clinical neurophysiology* (14th ed., Part 8). Amsterdam: Elsevier Scientific.

Courville, C. B. (1965). Contrecoup injuries of the brain in infancy. *Archives of Surgery, 90,* 157-165.

Craft, A. W., Shaw, D. A., & Cartlidge, N. E. (1972). Head injuries in children. *British Medical Journal, 4,* 200-203.

Crawford, J. R. (in press). Estimation of premorbid intelligence: A review of recent developments. In J. R. Crawford, & D. M. Parker (Eds.), *Developments in clinical and experimental neuropsychology.* New York: Plenum.

Cullum, C. M., & Bigler, E. D. (1986). Ventricle size, cortical atrophy and the relationship with neuropsychological status in closed head injury: A quantitative analysis. *Journal of Clinical and Experimental Neuropsychology, 8,* 437-452.

Cusumano, S., Paolin, A., Di Paola, F., Boccaletto, F., Simini, G., Palermo, F., & Carteri, A. (1992). Assessing brain function in post-traumatic coma by means of bit-mapped SEPs, BAEPs, CT, SPET, and clinical scores. Prognostic implications. *Electroencephalography and Clinical Neurophysiology, 84,* 499-515.

Dacey, R. G., Alves, W. M., Rimel, R. W., Winn, R., & Jane, J. A. (1986). Neurosurgical complications after apparently minor head injury: Assessment of risk in a series of 610 patients. *Journal of Neurosurgery, 65,* 203-210.

Dennis, M. (1991). Frontal lobe function in childhood and adolescence: A heuristic for assessing attention regulation, executive control, and the intentional states important for social discourse. *Developmental Neuropsychology, 7,* 327-358.

Denny-Brown, D., & Russell, W. R. (1941). Experimental cerebral concussion. *Brain, 64,* 93-164.

Dimitrijevic, M. M., Dimitrijevic, M. R., Kinalski, R., McKay, W. B., & Sherwood, A. M. (1987). Neurophysiological assessment of motor disorders in patients with brain injury. In M. E. Minor, & K. A. Wagner (Eds.), *Neurotrauma: Treatment, rehabilitation and related issues No. 2* (pp. 81-88). Boston: Butterworths.

DiRocco, C., & Velardi, F. (1986). Epidemiology and etiology of craniocerebral trauma in the first two years of life. In A. J. Raimondi, M. Choux, & C. DiRocco (Eds.), *Head injuries in the newborn and infant* (pp. 125-139). New York: Springer-Verlag.

Duffy, F. H., & McAnulty, G. B. (1985). Brain electrical mapping (BEAM): The search for a physiological signature of dyslexia. In F. H. Duffy, & N. Geschwind (Eds.), *Dyslexia: A neuroscientific approach to clinical evaluation* (pp. 105-122). Boston: Little, Brown.

Edna, T. H. (1987). Head injuries admitted to hospital: Epidemiology, risk factors and long term outcome. *Journal of the Oslo City Hospitals, 37,* 101-116.

Eichelberger, M. R., & Ball, J. W. (1990). *EMSC: Assessment Battery for the Brain Injured Child.* Washington, DC: Children's Hospital National Medical Center.

Eisenberg, H. M., Levin, H. S., & Papanicolauo, A. C. (1985). Recovery of memory after head injury. In R. G. Dacey, Jr., R. R. Winn, R. W. Rimel, & J. A. Jane (Eds.), *Seminars in neurological surgery: Trauma of the central nervous system* (pp. 35-47). New York: Raven.

Esparza, J., M-Portillo, J., Sarabia, M., Yuste, J. A., Roger, R., & Lamas, E. (1985). Outcome in children with severe head injuries. *Child's Nervous System, 1,* 109-114.

Ewing-Cobbs, L., & Fletcher, J. M. (in press). Neurobehavioral outcome following traumatic brain injury in children and adolescents. *Current Opinion in Pediatrics.*

Ewing-Cobbs, L., Fletcher, J. M., & Levin, H. S. (1986). Neurobehavioral sequelae following head injury in children: Educational implications. *Journal of Head Trauma Rehabilitation, 1,* 57-65.

Ewing-Cobbs, L., Fletcher, J. M., Levin, H. S., Copeland, K., Francis, D., & Miner, M. (1994, February). *Closed head injury in infants and preschoolers: A three year longitudinal neuropsychological follow-up.* Paper presented at the Twenty-Second Annual Meeting of the International Neuropsychological Society, Cincinnati, OH.

Ewing-Cobbs, L., Fletcher, J. M., Levin, H. S., & Landry, S. H. (1985). Language disorders after pediatric head injury. In J. K. Darby (Ed.), *Speech and language evaluation in neurology: Childhood disorders* (pp. 97-112). Orlando, FL: Grune & Stratton.

Ewing-Cobbs, L., Levin, H. S., Eisenberg, H. M., & Fletcher, J. M. (1987). Language functions following closed head injury in children and adolescents. *Journal of Clinical and Experimental Neuropsychology, 9,* 575-592.

Ewing-Cobbs, L., Levin, H. S., Fletcher, J. M., Miner, M. E., & Eisenberg, H. M. (1990). The Children's Orientation and Amnesia Test: Relationship to severity of acute head injury and to recovery of memory. *Neurosurgery, 27,* 683-691.

Eyberg, S. M., & Robinson, E. A. (1983). Dyadic parent-child interaction coding system: A manual. *Psychological Documents, 13,* (Ms. No. 2582).

Fedio, P., & Mirsky, A. F. (1969). Selective intellectual deficits in children with temporal lobe or centrencephalic epilepsy. *Neuropsychologia, 7,* 287-300.

Fennell, E. B., & Mickle, J. P. (1992). Behavioral effects of head trauma in children and adolescents. In M. G. Tramontana & S. R. Hooper (Eds.), *Advances in child neuropsychology* (Vol. 1, pp. 24-49). New York: Springer-Verlag.

Field, J. H. (1976). *Epidemiology of head injury in England and Wales: With particular application to rehabilitation.* Leicester, UK: Willsons.

Filley, C. M., Cranberg, L. D., Alexander, M. P., & Hart, E. J. (1987). Neurobehavioral outcome after closed head injury in childhood and adolescence. *Archives of Neurology, 44,* 194-198.

Flach, J., & Malmros, R. (1972). A long-term follow-up study of children with severe head injury. *Scandinavian Journal of Rehabilitation Medicine, 4,* 9-15.

Fletcher, J. M., Ewing-Cobbs, L., McLaughlin, E. J., & Levin, H. S. (1985). Cognitive and psychosocial sequelae of head injury in children: Implications for assessment and management. In B. F. Brooks (Ed.), *The injured child* (pp. 30-39). Austin: University of Texas Press.

Fletcher, J. M., Ewing-Cobbs, L., Miner, M. E., Levin, H. S., & Eisenberg, H. M. (1990). Behavioral changes after closed head injury in children. *Journal of Consulting and Clinical Psychology, 58,* 93-98.

Fletcher, J. M., & Levin, H. S. (1988). Neurobehavioral effects of brain injury in children. In D. K. Routh (Ed.), *Handbook of pediatric psychology* (pp. 258-295). New York: Guilford.

Fletcher, J. M., Miner, M. E., & Ewing-Cobbs, L. (1987). Age and recovery from head injury in children: Developmental issues. In H. S. Levin, J. Grafman, & H. M. Eisenberg (Eds.), *Neurobehavioral recovery from head injury* (pp. 279-291). New York: Oxford University Press.

Fletcher, J. M., & Taylor, H. G. (1984). Neuropsychological approaches to children: Towards a developmental neuropsychology. *Journal of Clinical Neuropsychology, 6,* 39-56.

Forehand, R., & McMahon, R. J. (1981). *Helping the noncompliant child: A clinician's guide to parent training.* New York: Guilford.

Frankowski, R. F. (1985). Head injury mortality in urban populations and its relation to the injured child. In B. F. Brooks (Ed.), *The injured child* (pp. 20-29). Austin: University of Texas Press.

Frankowski, R. F., Annegers, J. F., & Whitman, S. (1985). Epidemiological and descriptive studies: Part I. The descriptive epidemiology of head trauma in the United States. In D. P. Becker, & J. T. Povlishock (Eds.), *Central nervous system trauma status report— 1985* (pp. 33-43). Bethesda, MD: National Institute of Neurological and Communicative Disorders and Stroke, National Institutes of Health.

Fuld, P. A., & Fisher, P. (1977). Recovery of intellectual ability after closed head injury. *Developmental Medicine and Child Neurology, 19,* 495-502.

Gaddes, W. H. (1985). *Learning disabilities and brain function. A neuropsychological approach* (2nd ed.). New York: Springer-Verlag.

Gennarelli, T. A. (1986). Mechanisms and pathophysiology of cerebral concussion. *Journal of Head Trauma Rehabilitation, 1,* 23-30.

Gentry, L. R., Godersky, J. C., Thompson, B., & Dunn, V. D. (1988). Prospective comparative study of intermediate-field MR and CT in the evaluation of closed head trauma. *American Journal of Radiology, 150,* 673-682.

Gilchrist, E., & Wilkinson, M. (1979). Some factors determining prognosis in young people with severe head injuries. *Archives of Neurology, 36,* 355-359.

Gilroy, J., & Meyer, J. S. (1979). *Medical neurology* (2nd ed.). New York: Macmillan.

Glang, A., Singer, G., Cooley, E., & Tish, N. (1992). Tailoring direct instruction techniques for use with elementary students with brain injury. *Journal of Head Trauma Rehabilitation, 7,* 93-108.

Goldstein, F. C., & Levin, H. S. (1987). Epidemiology of pediatric closed head injury: Incidence, clinical characteristics, and risk factors. *Journal of Learning Disabilities, 20,* 518-525.

Gomori, J. M., Grossman, R. I., & Goldberg, H. I. (1985). Intracranial hematomas: Imaging by high-field MR. *Radiology, 157,* 87-93.

Graham, D. I., Adams, J. H., & Gennarelli, T. A. (1987). Pathology of brain damage in head injury. In P. R. Cooper (Ed.), *Head injury* (pp. 72-88). Baltimore, MD: Williams & Wilkins.

Grand, W. (1974). The significance of post-traumatic status epilepticus in childhood. *Journal of Neurology, Neurosurgery, and Psychiatry, 37,* 178-180.

Gulbrandsen, G. B. (1984). Neuropsychological sequela of light head injuries in older children six months after trauma. *Journal of Clinical Neuropsychology, 6,* 257-268.

Guyer, B., & Ellers, B. (1990). Childhood injuries in the United States. *American Journal of Diseases of Children, 144,* 649-652.

Hahn, Y. S., Chyung, C., Barthel, M. J., Bailes, J., Flannery, A., & McLone, D. G. (1988). Head injuries in children under 36 months of age. *Child's Nervous System, 4,* 34-40.

Halperin, J. M., McKay, K. E., Matier, K., & Sharma, V. (1994). Attention response inhibition, and activity level in children: Developmental neuropsychological perspectives. In M. G. Tramontara & S. R. Hooper (Eds.), *Advances in child neuropsychology* (Vol. 2, pp. 1-54). New York: Springer-Verlag.

Hecaen, H. (1976). Acquired aphasia in children and the ontogenesis of hemispheric functional specialization. *Brain and Language, 3,* 114-134.

Heiden, J., Small, R., Canton, W., Weiss, M., & Kurtze, T. (1983). Severe head injury. *Journal of the American Physical Therapy Association, 63,* 4-9.

Heiskanen, D., & Kaste, M. (1974). Late prognosis of severe brain injury in children. *Developmental Medicine and Child Neurology, 16,* 11-14.

Heiskanen, O., & Sipponen, P. (1970). Prognosis of severe head injury. *Acta Neurologica Scandinavica, 46,* 343-350.

Hendrick, E. B., Harwood-Nash, D.C.F., & Hudson, A. R. (1963). Head injuries in children: A survey of 4465 consecutive cases at the Hospital for Sick Children, Toronto, Canada. *Clinical Neurosurgery, 11,* 46-65.

Hounsfield, G. N. (1973). Computerized transverse axial scanning (tomography): Part I. Description of system. *British Journal of Radiology, 46,* 1016.

Hynd, G. W., & Willis, W. G. (1988). *Pediatric neuropsychology.* Orlando, FL: Grune & Stratton.

Ito, U., Tomita, H., Yamazaki, S., Takada, Y., & Inaba, Y. (1986). Brain swelling and brain edema in acute head injury. *Acta Neurochiro, 79,* 120-124.

Ivan, L. F., Choo, S. H., & Ventureya, E. C. (1983). Head injuries in childhood: A 2 year survey. *Canadian Medical Association Journal, 128,* 281-284.

Jagger, J., Levine, J. I., Jane, J., & Rimel, R. W. (1984). Epidemiologic features of head injury in a predominantly rural population. *Journal of Trauma, 24,* 40-44.

Jennett, B. (1975). *Epilepsy after non-missile head injuries* (2nd ed.). London: William Heinemann Medical Books.

Jennett, B. (1986). Head trauma. In A. K. Asbury, G. M. McKhann, & W. I. McDonald (Eds.), *Diseases of the nervous system* (pp. 1282-1291). Philadelphia: W. B. Saunders.

Jennett, B., & Teasdale, G. (1981). *Management of head injuries.* Philadelphia: F. A. Davis.

Jordon, F. M., Ozanne, A. E., & Murdoch, B. E. (1990). Performance of closed head injured children on a naming task. *Brain Injury, 4,* 27-32.

Kaiser, G., & Pfenninger, J. (1984). Effect of neurointensive care upon outcome following severe head injuries in childhood: A preliminary report. *Neuropediatrics, 15,* 68-75.

Kalsbeek, W. D., McLaurin, R. L., Harris, B. S., & Miller, J. D. (1980). The national head and spinal cord injury survey: Major findings. *Journal of Neurosurgery, 53,* 19-31.

Kampen, D. L., & Grafman, J. (1989). Neuropsychological evaluation of penetrating head injury. In M. D. Lezak (Ed.), *Assessment of the behavioral consequences of head trauma* (pp. 49-60). New York: Alan R. Liss.

Kang, J. K., Park, C. K., Kim, M. C., Kim, D. S., & Song, J. U. (1989). Traumatic isolated intracerebral hemorrhage in children. *Child's Nervous System, 5,* 303-306.

Kaplan, E., Fein, D., Morris, R., & Delis, D. C. (1991). *WAIS-R as a neuropsychological instrument.* San Antonio: The Psychological Corporation.

Kaufman, A. S., & Kaufman, N. L. (1990). *Kaufman Brief Intelligence Test.* Circle Pines, MN: American Guidance Service.

Kaufman, H. H., Makela, M. E., Lee, K. F., Haid, R. W., Jr., & Gildenberg, P. L. (1986). Gunshot wounds to the head: A perspective. *Neurosurgery, 18,* 689-695.

Kazdin, A. E. (1988). *Child psychotherapy: Developing and identifying effective treatment.* New York: Pergamon.

Kazdin, A. E. (1993). Psychotherapy for children and adolescents: Current progress and future directions. *American Psychologist, 48,* 644-657.

Klauber, M. R., Barrett-Connor, E., Marshall, L. F., & Bowers, S. A. (1981). The epidemiology of head injury: A prospective study of an entire community—San Diego County, California, 1978. *American Journal of Epidemiology, 113,* 500-509.

Klonoff, H. (1971). Head injuries in children: Predisposing factors, accident conditions, accident proneness and sequelae. *American Journal of Public Health, 61,* 2405-2417.

Klonoff, H., Low, M. D., & Clark, D. (1977). Head injuries in children: A prospective five-year follow-up. *Journal of Neurology, Neurosurgery, and Psychiatry, 40,* 1211-1219.

Klonoff, H., & Paris, R. (1974). Immediate, short-term and residual effects of acute head injuries in children: Neuropsychological and neurological correlates. In R. M. Reitan, & L. A. Davison (Eds.), *Clinical neuropsychology: Current status and applications* (pp. 179-219). New York: John Wiley.

Klonoff, H., & Thompson, G. B. (1969). Epidemiology of head injuries in adults: A pilot study. *Canadian Medical Association Journal, 100,* 235-241.

Kraus, J. F. (1987). Epidemiology of head injury. In P. R. Cooper (Ed.), *Head injury* (2nd ed., pp. 1-19). Baltimore, MD: Williams & Wilkins.

Kraus, J. F., Black, M. A., Hessol, N., Ley, P., Rokaw, W., Sullivan, C., Bowers, S., Knowlton, S., & Marshall, L. (1984). The incidence of acute brain injury and serious impairment in a defined population. *American Journal of Epidemiology, 119,* 186-201.

Kraus, J. F., Fife, D., Cox, P., Ramstein, K., & Conroy, C. (1986). Incidence, severity, and external causes of pediatric brain injury. *American Journal of Diseases of Children, 140,* 687-693.

Kraus, J. F., Rock, A., & Hemyari, P. (1990). Brain injuries among infants, children, adolescents, and young adults. *American Journal of Diseases of Children, 144,* 684-691.

Lange-Cosack, H., Wider, B., Schlesner, H. J., Grumme, T., & Kubicki, S. (1979). Prognosis of brain injuries in young children (one until five years of age). *Neuropadiatrie, 10,* 105-127.

Lanser, J. B., Jennekens-Schinkel, A., & Peters, A. C. (1988). Headache after closed head injury in children. *Headache, 28,* 176-179.

Levin, A. V., Magnusson, M. R., Rafto, S. E., & Zimmerman, R. A. (1989). Shaken baby syndrome diagnosed by magnetic resonance imaging. *Pediatric Emergency Care, 5,* 181-186.

Levin, H. S., & Benton, A. L. (1986). Developmental and acquired dyscalculia in children. In I. Flehmig & L. Stern (Eds.), *Child development and learning behavior* (pp. 317-322). Stuttgart: Guustav Fisher.

Levin, H. S., & Eisenberg, H. M. (1979a). Neuropsychological impairment after closed head injury in children and adolescents. *Journal of Pediatric Psychology, 4,* 389-402.

Levin, H. S., & Eisenberg, H. M. (1979b). Neuropsychological outcome of closed head injury in children and adolescents. *Child's Brain, 5,* 281-292.

Levin, H. S., Eisenberg, H. M., Wigg, N. R., & Kobayashi, K. (1982). Memory and intellectual ability after head injury in children and adolescents. *Neurosurgery, 11,* 668-673.

Levin, H. S., High, W. M., Ewing-Cobbs, L., Fletcher, J. M., Eisenberg, H. M., Miner, M. E., & Goldstein, F. C. (1988). Memory functioning during the first year after closed head injury in children and adolescents. *Neurosurgery, 22,* 1043-1052.

Levin, H. S., Meyers, C. A., Grossman, R. G., & Sarwar, M. (1981). Ventricular enlargement after closed head injury. *Archives of Neurology, 38,* 623-629.

Levin, H. S., O'Donnell, V. M., & Grossman, R. G. (1979). The Galveston Orientation and Amnesia Test: A practical scale to assess cognition after head injury. *Journal of Nervous and Mental Disease, 167,* 675-684.

Lezak, M. D. (1983). *Neuropsychological assessment* (2nd ed.). New York: Oxford University Press.

Lieh-Lai, M. W., Theodorou, A. A., Sarnaik, A. P., Meert, K. L., Moylan, P. M., & Canady, A. I. (1992). Limitations of the Glasgow Coma Scale in predicting outcome in children with traumatic brain injury. *Journal of Pediatrics, 120,* 195-199.

Lindenberg, R., & Freytag, E. (1960). The mechanism of cerebral contusions. *Archives of Pathology, 69,* 440-469.

Lipper, M. H., Kishore, P. R., Enas, G. G., Domingues-da-Silva, A. A., Choi, S. C., & Becker, D. P. (1985). Computed tomography in the prediction of outcome in head injury. *American Journal of Radiology, 144,* 483-486.

Luria, A. R. (1966). *Human brain and psychological process.* New York: Harper & Row.

Mahoney, W. J., D'Souza, B. J., Haller, A., Rogers, M. D., Epstein, M. H., & Freeman, J. M. (1983). Long-term outcome of children with severe head trauma and prolonged coma. *Pediatrics, 71,* 756-762.

Martin, D. A. (1990). Family issues in traumatic brain injury. In E. D. Bigler (Ed.), *Traumatic brain injury. Mechanisms of damage, assessment, intervention, and outcome* (pp. 381-394). Austin, TX: Pro-Ed.

Martin, R. P., Hooper, S. R., & Snow, J. (1986). Behavior rating scale approaches to personality assessment in children and adolescents. In H. M. Knoff (Ed.), *The psychological assessment of child and adolescent personality* (pp. 309-351). New York: Guilford.

Mateer, C. A., & Williams, D. (1991). Effects of frontal lobe injury in childhood. *Developmental Neuropsychology, 7,* 359-376.

Mayes, S. D., Pelco, L. E., & Campbell, C. J. (1989). Relationships among pre- and post-injury intelligence, length of coma, and age in individuals with severe closed head injuries. *Brain Injury, 3,* 301-313.

McKissock, W., Richardson, A., & Bloom, W. H., (1960). Subdural hematoma. A review of 389 cases. *Lancet, 228,* 1365-1369.

Mealey, J. (1968). *Pediatric head injuries.* Springfield, IL: Charles C Thomas.

Menkes, J. H. (Ed.). (1985). *Textbook of child neurology* (3rd ed.). Philadelphia: Lea & Febiger.

Menkes, J. H. (Ed.). (1990). *Textbook of child neurology* (4th ed.). Philadelphia: Lea & Febiger.

Menkes, J. H., & Batzdorf, U. (1985). Postnatal trauma and injuries by physical agents. In J. H. Menkes (Ed.), *Textbook of child neurology* (3rd ed., pp. 471-505). Philadelphia: Lea & Febiger.

Michaud, L. J., Rivara, F. P., Jaffe, K. M., Fay, G., & Dailey, J. L. (1993). Traumatic brain injury as a risk factor for behavioral disorders in children. *Archives of Physical Medicine and Rehabilitation, 74,* 368-375.

Mills, M. L. (1986). High-yield criteria for urgent cranial computed tomography scans. *Annals of Emergency Medicine, 15,* 1167.

Mizrahi, E. M., & Kellaway, P. (1984). Cerebral concussion in children: Assessment of injury by electroencephalography. *Pediatrics, 73,* 419.

Morray, J. P., Tyler, D. C., Jones, T. K., Stunz, J. T., & Lemire, R. J. (1984). Coma scale for use in brain-injured children. *Critical Care Medicine, 12,* 1018-1020.

Moyes, C. D. (1980). Epidemiology of serious head injuries in childhood. *Child Care Health Development, 6,* 1-6.

Naglieri, J. A. (1985). *Matrix Analogies Test Expanded Form.* New York: Psychological Corporation.

National Head Injury Foundation. (1985). *An educator's manual: What educators need to know about students with traumatic brain injury.* Framingham, MA: Author.

North, A. F. (1976). When should a child be in the hospital? *Pediatrics, 57,* 540-543.

Ommaya, A. K., Grubbs, R. L., & Naumann, R. (1971). Coup and contrecoup injury: Observations on the mechanics of visible injuries in the rhesus monkey. *Journal of Neurosurgery, 35,* 503-516.

Pang, D. (1985). Pathophysiologic correlates of neurobehavioral syndromes following closed head injury. In M. Ylvisaker (Ed.), *Head injury rehabilitation: Children and adolescents* (pp. 3-70). San Diego, CA: College-Hill Press.

Patterson, G. R., & Bank, L. (1986). Bootstrapping your way in the nomological thicket. *Behavioral Assessment, 8,* 49-73.

Patterson, G. R., Ray, R. S., Shaw, D. A., & Cobb, J. A. (1969). *Manual for coding of family interactions* (rev. ed.). New York: Microfiche Publications.

Reitan, R. M., & Wolfson, D. (1985). *Neuroanatomy and neuropathology. A clinical guide for neuropsychologists.* Tucson, AZ: Neuropsychology Press.

Reynolds, C. R., & Gutkin, T. B. (1979). Predicting the premorbid intellectual status of children using demographic data. *Clinical Neuropsychology, 1,* 36-38.

Reynolds, C. R., & Richmond, B. O. (1985). *Revised Children's Manifest Anxiety Scale (RCMAS).* Los Angeles: Western Psychological Services.

Reynolds, W. M. (1987). *Reynolds Adolescent Depression Scale.* Odessa, FL: Psychological Assessment Resources.

Reynolds, W. M. (1989). *Reynolds Child Depression Scale.* Odessa, FL: Psychological Assessment Resources.

Rhawn, J. (1982). The neuropsychology of development: Hemispheric laterality, limbic language, and the origin of thought. *Journal of Clinical Psychology, 38,* 4-33.

Richardson, F. (1963). Some effects of severe head injury. A follow-up study of children and adolescents after protracted coma. *Developmental Medicine and Child Neurology, 5,* 471-482.

Rivara, F. P. (1984). Childhood injuries: III. Epidemiology of non-motor vehicle head trauma. *Developmental Medicine and Child Neurology, 26,* 81-87.

Rivara, F. P., & Mueller, B. A. (1986). The epidemiology and prevention of pediatric head injury. *Journal of Head Trauma Rehabilitation, 1,* 7-15.

Roberts, A. (1979). *Severe accidental head injury.* New York: Macmillian.

Rodin, E. A., Schmaltz, S., & Twitty, G. (1986). Intellectual functions of patients with childhood-onset epilepsy. *Developmental Medicine and Child Neurology, 28,* 25-33.

Rosen, C. D., & Gerring, J. P. (1986). *Head trauma: Educational reintegration.* San Diego, CA: College-Hill Press.

Rothenberger, A. (1986). Aphasia in children. *Fortschritte der Neurologic Psychiatric, 54,* 92-98.

Rourke, B. P., Bakker, D. J., Fisk, J. L., & Strang, J. D. (1983). *Child neuropsychology: An introduction to theory, research, and clinical practice.* New York: Guilford.

Rourke, B. P., Fisk, J. L., & Strang, J. D. (1986). *Neuropsychological assessment of children: A treatment-oriented approach.* New York: Guilford.

Ruff, R. M., Levin, H. S., Maltis, S., High, H. M., Marshall, L. F., Eisenberg, H. M., & Tobaddor, K. (1989). Recovery of memory after mild head injury: A three-center study. In H. S. Levin, H. M. Eisenberg, & A. L. Benton (Eds.), *Mild head injury* (pp. 176-188). New York: Oxford University Press.

Russell, W. R. (1971). *The traumatic amnesias.* London: Oxford University Press.

Rutter, M. (1981). Psychological sequelae of brain damage in children. *American Journal of Psychiatry, 138,* 1533-1544.

Rutter, M., Chadwick, O., Shaffer, D., & Brown, G. (1980). A prospective study of children with head injuries: 1. Design and methods. *Psychological Medicine, 10,* 633-645.

Salazar, A. M., Grafman, J., Schlesselman, S., Vance, S. C., Mohr, J. P., Carpenter, M., Pevsner, P., Ludlow, C., & Weingartner, H. (1986). Penetrating war injuries of the basal forebrain: Neurology and cognition. *Neurology, 36,* 459-465.

Sato, Y., Yuh, W. T. C., Smith, W. L., Alexander, R. C., Kao, S. C. S., & Ellerbrock, C. J. (1989). Head injury in child abuse: Evaluation with MR imaging. *Pediatric Radiology, 173,* 653-657.

Satz, P. (1993). Brain reserve capacity on symptom onset after brain injury: A formulation and review of evidence for threshold theory. *Neuropsychology, 7,* 273-295.

Savage, R. C. (1991). Identification, classification, and placement issues for students with traumatic brain injuries. *Journal of Head Trauma Rehabilitation, 6,* 1-9.

Schoenhuber, R., & Gentilini, M. (1986). Auditory brain stem responses in the prognosis of late postconcussional symptoms and neuropsychological dysfunction after minor head injury. *Neurosurgery, 19,* 532-534.

Sganzerla, E. P., Tomei, G., Guerra, P., Tiberio, F., Rampini, P. M., Gaini, S. M., & Villani, R. M. (1989). Clinicoradiological and therapeutic considerations in severe diffuse traumatic brain injury in children. *Child's Nervous System, 5,* 168-171.

Shaffer, D., Bijur, P., Chadwick, O. F. D., & Rutter, M. L. (1980). Head injury and later reading disability. *Journal of the American Academy of Child Psychiatry, 19,* 592-610.

Shapiro, K. (1987). Special considerations for the pediatric age group. In P. R. Cooper (Ed.), *Head injury* (pp. 367-389). Baltimore, MD: Williams & Wilkins.

Shurtleff, H., Abbott, R., Townes, B., & Berniger, V. (1990, August). *Structural equation modeling of neurodevelopmental, intellectual, and academic factors.* Paper presented at the Annual Meeting of the American Psychological Association, Boston.

Simpson, D., & Reilly, P. (1982). Pediatric coma scale. *Lancet, 2,* 450.

Slater, E. J., & Bassett, S. S. (1988). Adolescents with closed head injuries. *American Journal of Diseases of Children, 142,* 1048-1051.

Snow, J. H. (in press). Executive functions with different pediatric groups. *International Journal of Clinical Neuropsychology.*

Soloniuk, D., Pitts, L. H., Lovely, M., & Bartkowski, H. (1986). Traumatic intracerebral hematomas: Timing of appearance and indications for operative removal. *Journal of Trauma, 26,* 787-794.

Spatz, H. (1950). Brain injuries in aviation in German aviation medicine World War II. *Department of the Air Force, 1,* 616-640.

Spielberger, C. D. (1988). *State-Trait Anger Expression Inventory* (research ed.). Odessa, FL: Psychological Assessment Resources.

Spreen, O., & Gaddes, W. H. (1969). Developmental norms for 15 neuropsychological tests ages 6-16. *Cortex, 5,* 171-191.

Spreen, O., & Straus, E. (1991). *A compendium of neuropsychological tests: Administration, norms, and commentary.* New York: Oxford University Press.

Spreen, O., Tupper, D., Risser, A., Tuokko, H., & Edgell, D. (1984). *Human developmental neuropsychology.* New York: Oxford University Press.

Stevens, C. F. (1979). The neuron. *Scientific American, 241,* 54-65.

Stuss, D. T., & Berson, D. F. (1986). *The frontal lobes.* New York: Raven Press.

Taylor, H. G. (1984). Early brain injury and cognitive development. In C. R. Almli & S. Finger (Eds.), *Early brain injury* (pp. 325-341). New York: Academic Press.

Teasdale, G., & Jennett, B. (1974). Assessment of coma and impaired consciousness. A practical scale. *Lancet, 2,* 81-84.

U.S. Office of Education (1992). Individuals with Disabilities Education Act (IDEA). *Federal Register, 57 (189),* 44842-44843.

Wahler, R. G., House, A. E., & Stambaugh, E. E. (1976). *Ecological assessment of child problem behavior: A clinical package for home, school, and institutional settings.* New York: Pergamon.

Watson, P. J. (1978). Nonmotor functions of the cerebellum. *Psychological Bulletin, 85,* 944-967.

Wechsler, D. (1974). *Manual for the Wechsler Intelligence Scale for Children-Revised.* San Antonio, TX: The Psychological Corporation.

Winogron, H. W., Knights, R. M., & Bawden, H. N. (1984). Neuropsychological deficits following head injury in children. *Journal of Clinical Neuropsychology, 6,* 269-286.

Ylvisaker, M. (1986). Language and communication disorders following pediatric head injury. *Journal of Head Trauma Rehabilitation, 1,* 48-56.

Ylvisaker, M., Hartwick, P., & Stevens, M. (1991). School reentry following head injury: Managing the transition from hospital to school. *Journal of Head Trauma Rehabilitation, 6,* 10-22.

Yoshino, E., Yamaki, T., Higuchi, T., Horikawa, Y., & Hirakawa, K. (1985). Acute brain edema in fatal head injury: Analysis by dynamic CT scanning. *Journal of Neurosurgery, 63,* 830-839.

Index

ABOUT THE AUTHORS

Jeffrey H. Snow is Neuropsychologist for the Nevada Community Enrichment Program. He is a member of the editorial advisory boards for the *Journal of Psychoeducational Assessment* and *Assessment in Rehabilitation and Exceptionality* and has published numerous articles in the area of developmental neuropsychology. He holds a Diplomate in Clinical Neuropsychology from the American Board of Professional Psychology.

Stephen R. Hooper is Psychology Section Head and Director of Child and Adolescent Neuropsychology at the Clinical Center for the Study of Development and Learning of the Child Development Institute at the University of North Carolina School of Medicine as well as Associate Professor in the Department of Psychiatry at the University of North Carolina School of Medicine, Clinical Assistant Professor in the School of Education, and Research Assistant Professor in the Department of Psychology at the University of North Carolina at Chapel Hill. He is a member of the editorial advisory boards for *Developmental Neuropsychology,* the *Journal of Clinical Child Psychology,* and the *Journal of Psychoeducational Assessment,* and he reviews regularly for other major journals in the fields of school psychology, clinical psychology, and neuropsychology. He is widely published in the areas of child neuropsychology and child psychopathology. He is coeditor of the series *Advances in Child Neuropsychology* and of the forthcoming series *Topics in Child Neuropsychology.* His most recent books include *Assessment and Diagnosis of Child and Adolescent Psychopathology* and *The Neurological Basis of Child Psychopathology.*